THE STATE OF MEDICINE

THE STATE
OF MEDICINE

A Critical Review

by

John W. Todd

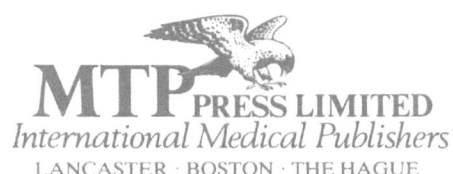

MTP PRESS LIMITED
International Medical Publishers
LANCASTER · BOSTON · THE HAGUE

Published by
MTP Press Limited
Falcon House
Lancaster, England

ISBN-13: 978-94-011-7247-9   e-ISBN-13: 978-94-011-7245-5
DOI: 10.1007/ 978-94-011-7245-5

Phototypesetting by Art Associates, (Manchester) Ltd.

Contents

Acknowledgments

I am delighted to thank the following: my sons, Peter and Charles, both doctors, who read the entire typescript, corrected errors and made many useful suggestions. Dr David Ryde (who has shown that a General Practitioner can be popular and successful while having prescription costs around one-fifth of the national average). He too read the typescript and gave me valuable advice. My wife, who read the proofs and noted many errors.

John W. Todd,
Farnham, Surrey

Preface

As a young general practitioner new to the field I recall how stimulated and excited I was by reading Dr John W. Todd's papers in the *Lancet* some 20–30 years ago. It was as though a lot of dust had been blown away and I was able for once to see the situation of medicine much more clearly.

He became one of my medical heroes to add to John Ryle, Henry Cohen and René Dubois – all of whom have influenced my own approach to medical care and caring of my patients.

Now in 1981, it is a pleasure to write an introductory foreword to this book.

The *State of Medicine* represents the clear and honest thoughts of a most unusual person. Until his retirement John W. Todd was a general physician in Farnham, Surrey. He was relatively unknown to the medical profession outside Surrey apart from his occasional writings.

The ten chapters show the build-up of wide experience and deep philosophy that accumulated during his years in practice.

I find that I am as stimulated and excited now reading them, as I was 20–30 years ago. I may not agree with all that he writes and others likewise may disagree completely – but I commend the work as an invigorating experience.

John Fry,
Beckenham, Kent

1

Medical Education

In so far as doctors have mistaken attitudes towards the problems of medicine these must be attributed in part to their education. This has been a favourite topic for debate for many years. Everyone agrees that students are taught the wrong things in the wrong way, but there is an almost total lack of agreement as to what reforms are needed.

Every critic tends to grind his own axe. Most patients are old; therefore more time should be devoted to geriatrics. Next to the old, many patients are babies and young children and therefore more time should be devoted to paediatrics. More hours are lost from work on account of the rheumatic complaints than from the other group of maladies; therefore more should be learnt about rheumatism. The amount of psychiatric illness is immense; therefore students should spend longer in studying this kind of illness. Prevention is better than cure but doctors traditionally wait until patients have 'established disease'; therefore students should be taught to get among the populace and prevent them from ever becoming ill. More women than men visit the doctor, but the medical profession is male orientated and doctors don't take women's problems seriously; therefore they should be taught how to take them seriously. And so on.

Is it possible to reach any objective conclusions among all these

1

disparate voices? I shall attempt to answer this difficult question in the present chapter.

EDUCATION BEFORE MEDICAL SCHOOL

Before the Second World War many students arrived at their medical schools having studied humanities in their sixth forms. They then spent a year doing physics, chemistry, and biology for their first MB examinations, whereas now nearly all students have spent their 2 or 3 years in the sixth form largely studying these subjects. The decision that they will become doctors has therefore effectively been made when they were only 16 years old, or even younger. In consequence, it has been alleged, they start their medical education already narrow specialists, sometimes hardly able to write a decent sentence, and almost totally ignorant of the outside world. To what extent is this true? And in so far as it is true, do these students in consequence become worse doctors?

Whether or not a narrow early education makes students into worse doctors, a broad education is intrinsically desirable. The ability to express one's thoughts on paper and to write good English is, moreover, of practical value in everyday life. The mature adult who knows something of history and literature, who is aware of the problems of the Third World, and who can speak and write another language than his own is a 'better' citizen than is the one who lacks this knowledge.

Should all schoolchildren, therefore, have a broad education until they leave school and only specialize when they reach the university? And should medical students do a broad course in their first years at university, as they do in the United States and to some extent at Oxford and Cambridge? The London medical schools, which produce so many British doctors, are exceptional in that they are physically separate from the other parts of London University. London clinical students, therefore, do not mix with other students in common-rooms, dining rooms and clubs, as they do at Oxford and Cambridge and at the Scottish and English provincial medical schools. How much does this encourage a narrow outlook?

Objective answers cannot be given to questions of this kind. Whether or not later specialization would produce more rounded citizens and better doctors, it has the great disadvantage of prolonging an already long medical course. Most young people have a strong desire for independence and to be earning their own living, and often feel frustrated that for so long they are dependent upon grants and upon their parents. Their frustration would be even worse if they had to spend several more years before they qualified. The separation of medical students from other students which occurs in London seems to me undesirable, though whether in practice it has appreciable ill effects it is impossible to say.

Looking back at my student days, some of my fellow students did seem exclusively preoccupied by their medical studies, whereas others found plenty of time for outside interests. I recall a student who won numerous prizes and never failed an exam but who appeared astonishingly ignorant of everything outside medicine and sport.

A young person's interests do not just depend on his education at school or university. They are also largely influenced by the family background. If, throughout his early years, a child lives in a home filled with intellectual activity on a broad front he will probably continue to have broad interests, even if he does specialize in chemistry, physics, and biology as soon as he has taken his O level exams. And for the rest of his life he may continue to believe that education in its widest sense is a lifelong process.

Chemistry is a most important basic science. Without it biochemistry cannot be understood, and some awareness of biochemistry is essential to the doctor. Physics cannot be closely related to medicine except in the fields of radiology and radiotherapy. A knowledge of biology as a whole should be part of any liberal education. There is no apparent reason why medical students should know more biology than do other students. In the past botany was an important part of the medical curriculum because the doctor had to make his own medicines from plants, but this has long been irrelevant.

THE PRECLINICAL PERIOD AT MEDICAL SCHOOL

For generations medical students in Britain have spent some 2 years mainly studying anatomy, including normal histology, and physiology, including biochemistry, before they have begun to learn about sick people. Without doubt this grounding is sound in principle, though there is endless debate about details.

To most people anatomy is the dullest of all dull subjects. It is exceptional among sciences in that there cannot be any more important discoveries to be made about it. Although new editions of textbooks of anatomy continue to appear, the student can manage quite well with an edition of 100 years ago. There are no great underlying principles to be learnt and the student just has to memorize in turn the various structures in the various parts of the body.

Notoriously, students start to forget their anatomy as soon as they have passed their exams, and after a few years not much remains. Surgeons of course retain a knowledge of the anatomy of that region in which they specialize, but they forget most of the remainder. It is difficult to argue that this loss matters a great deal. Students should, therefore, spend less time on anatomy than has been the custom in the past. On the other hand, if students learn only a sketchy outline, they will still forget most of what they are taught and in the end will retain hardly any. To reach a firm conclusion on this difficult problem is hardly possible.

No doubt anatomy is made less dull if its practical applications to medicine and surgery are pointed out to the students. Some teachers attempt to do this, and there are also sections devoted to 'applied anatomy' in some textbooks. Unfortunately, many teachers succeed in making an already dull subject even duller.

Physiology, including biochemistry, is the supremely important basic science for the doctor. Its study should give the student an understanding both of how the bodily organs work and of scientific method. Of course, a great deal of physiology is forgotten. But, whereas for most doctors forgetting anatomy rarely matters, and whereas on the uncommon occasions in the doctor's life when some anatomical point is relevant a book can be consulted, the doctor who forgets all his physiology must make mistakes. An awareness of the digestive process, of the autonomic nervous system, of the workings of the liver and kidneys, and of the endocrine glands and their interrelationships often influences — or should influence — clinical decisions.

In particular, pharmacology is largely dependent on physiology.

Without physiology, pharmacology can be little more than learning parrot-wise about the effects of drugs. On the other hand, pharmacology is very much applied science. A drug is not proved to be valuable because it is shown in the laboratory to have a certain effect; the final test of a drug is the empirical test that it works in practice. During the war there were many cases of secondary 'shock' following upon crush injuries and the victims produced little or no urine. They were given sodium sulphate intravenously because it was deduced that the sulphate ion, as it is not reabsorbed in the kidney tubules, *must* take with it a quantity of water, and re-establish the urinary flow. Unfortunately, this theoretical edifice was not accompanied by any such effect in practice. Metaraminol, though less popular than it was, is still recommended for patients in 'shock' because it raises the blood pressure. It is assumed that this *must* be beneficial but there is no firm evidence that in practice metaraminol saves life. Digoxin is given to patients with cardiac failure in normal sinus rhythm largely because of experiments in the laboratory about the effect of digoxin on isolated animal's hearts. In spite of the fact that digitalis has been in use over 200 years, there is no clear proof that it is effective in this situation.

The preclinical medical student should also learn something about psychology. The development of the child's personality, the meaning of such concepts as intelligence and character, and the validity of various psychological tests are of general interest. He should also learn about the various theories of psychology, and in particular the Freudian and its offshoots. But whereas a knowledge of anatomy and physiology is an essential prerequisite to the understanding of bodily disease, one may doubt whether a course on academic psychology helps much in understanding the nature and varieties of mental disorder.

THE CLINICAL PERIOD

Several times in this book I suggest that a prime medical error is to concentrate the attention on the particular region of which the patient is complaining and to fail to look at him as a whole person. All kinds of doctors are liable to make this error, but the worst offenders tend to be the ultra-specialists, for obvious reasons.

Students who are taught by those with this approach are naturally liable to develop the same approach when they go out into the world. When faced by a patient with, say, headache, they will think of all the 'organic' possibilities — sinusitis, refractive error, cerebral tumour, cervical spondylopathy, hypertension etc. — but never sit back and look at the patient as a whole. They may do various investigations and refer the patient to various specialists. Whereas if they had just talked to the patient about his headache, his background, and his worries, it would have been evident that his head sensations reflected his emotional state.

How can we break this vicious circle of error? There is no easy answer here. We can only hope that the widespread condemnation of this narrow attitude will in time put things right. The situation is better than it was some 50 years ago, during the worst of the mechanistic age of medicine. At least, we do not now pleat the stomachs or fix the kidneys of neurotic women with chronic abdominal symptoms.

However extreme are the disagreements about the medical curriculum, no-one disputes the principle that medical students, like other students, should be encouraged to think for themselves. And we all agree that this ability is a necessary attribute of the educated man. But there has been far too great a tendency, not to educate, but to instruct medical students.

G.W. Pickering[1], who was the Regius Professor of Medicine at Oxford University, commented that a colleague of his who taught English told him that 'medical students were not being educated, they were being instructed . He explained that education was a training of the mind. The process of instruction, on the other hand, was a process of forced feeding, in which nothing was required of the student except to memorize and to reproduce what he remembered. In such a process the student was required to know the conclusions but not necessarily the evidence on which these were based'. Pickering continued, 'It was clear to me that he was right, and this became even clearer to me in the clinical years, when many teachers did not themselves know what the evidence was or where it could be found'.

My memories of my medical education are similar to those of Pickering's. When studying physiology Professor Samson Wright and his colleagues did encourage the students to think for themselves, to ask questions and to argue. But the eminent physicians and surgeons who taught me were too fond of making *ex cathedra* pronouncements. Many were consciously Great Men who did not demean themselves by arguing with mere students. Especially in the field of treatment were they highly uncritical. I recall the Senior Physician, who was invariably courteous to patients, students and nurses alike, saying of some remedy (which everyone would now accept is entirely valueless): 'I am sure it does good, dear boy'. No student would have dared to question this statement. We were often told, or it was taken for granted, that the Great Man's experience had proved that some remedy was useful. The Great Man did not tell us that experience could be most misleading, that we should always bear in mind the *post hoc ergo propter hoc* fallacy, and that most patients recover from most illnesses with the aid of Nature alone. Our teachers failed, as do many of their successors today, to distinguish between treatment based on theory and treatment based on evidence.

Rest was the almost universal remedy, after operations and childbirth, for all feverish illnesses, and in particular for tuberculosis, coronary thrombosis and congestive heart failure, rheumatic fever, and peptic ulcer. The theoretical grounds for advocating it seemed so overwhelmingly strong that virtually no-one doubted its value. And no-one pointed out that the only way of determining whether or not rest was beneficial was to compare a group of patients who were rested with another group who were not.

In the 17th century the powerful Paris faculty issued a decree that 'none may deviate from Hippocrates or Galen upon pain of excommunication'. And until the early 19th century it was taken for granted that anything said by Galen was true. In my student days we had advanced beyond this. Since then we have advanced further still. Few teaching hospital consultants now adopt that mantle of infallibility which too many of them adopted in my student days. Today's medical students are less cowed than we were and less likely to accept the Great Man's dictum as inspired truth. Few consultants would defend their action on the ground that 'my experience proves it to be true', and if they did the students would deride them behind their backs. But there nevertheless probably remains a tendency to instruct rather than to educate.

Medical students are still not always encouraged to be critical of theories of aetiology, of concepts of disease, and in particular, of treatment. Students should constantly ask questions of the following kind. This patient has been ordered 'physiotherapy'; what does this mean and in what way will it help? Why has the patient been kept in bed? How would he have been harmed if he had been allowed up? This patient is to have 'formal psychotherapy'; what good will that do? Is there any evidence that speech therapy will hasten the recovery of this aphasic patient? Why should this patient be in hospital at all? He has a good home, so would it not be better for all concerned if he stayed there? One may suspect that students who did ask such questions would often be given short shrift.

These attitudes which I am condemning are sometimes defended on the ground that medicine, unlike other scientific subjects, is an Art as well as a science. This has been believed for a long time. In 1871 Dr Alfred Stille said in his presidential address to the American Medical Association: 'Science does its full share of work for medicine; for no other art does it do so much. But we err greatly if we accept it as a certain and sole guide... A physician in the highest sense is an artist whom no amount of knowledge and no degree of culture can ever elevate to a high rank in his profession unless he has the perception of form, colour, proportion, and the manifold qualities and relations of things, which is a gift of genius as certainly as the poet's, the painter's, the sculptor's, or the architect's artistic eye'. Porritt (1960) in his presidential address[2] to the British Medical Association, said: 'In ... surgery a major revolution has taken place in the last 20 years ... in the very drama of this intensely stimulating scene there is the danger at times of forgetting the central figure — the patient. For medicine is still an art as well as a science. Has the art deteriorated in the presence of the efflorescence of the science? Does the art still sufficiently control and assess the science in the light of the personal problems of the patient?'. According to Lawrence[3] (1950) the art of medicine 'mainly implies a humane and kindly consideration of our patients, an appreciation of their fears, their family ties, their social difficulties'. In an annotation in the *Practitioner* (1959)[4] we were told: 'in the diagnosis of the acute abdomen the art of medicine still reigns supreme .... No X-rays! No lab reports! No registrars or house-surgeons! Just the doctor on his own while time seems to stand still and the family waits on his verdict!'. And we were told by Collier (1950)[5] that: 'The dividing line that separates the art from the science of diagnosis falls roughly where symptoms begin to merge into the objective signs of illness and disease. So long as there are symptoms of illness but no discoverable physical signs, diagnosis, prognosis and treatment must be carried out by "art" and not by "science"'.

The 'art' of medicine is thus variously held to imply a perception of form, colour, proportion, and the manifold relation of things, the ability to remember the patient, a humane and kindly attitude, the ability to reach a diagnosis without investigations, and the interpretation of symptoms (as opposed to physical signs). It is indeed important to look at the patient as a whole, as I repeatedly conclude throughout this book. This seems to imply that to forget the patient and concentrate on the separate bits of his body is a scientific attitude. This is absurd. To fail to look at the patient is blind folly. Why should this be called science? Of course, doctors should be humane and kindly; this is civilized behaviour; why should it be called art? Reaching a diagnosis without investigations requires just the qualities as doing this with investigations. And sometimes the first is simple and the second difficult. Why should the one be called art and the other science? Interpreting symptoms can be simple. Why is it art? Interpreting physical signs can be a most subtle and difficult matter. Why should it be called science?

This idea that the practice of medicine encompasses the two antitheses science and art is, then, false. It also implies an obscurantist approach. And it does not justify the view that the problems of medicine should be looked at in a less critical way than the problems of other disciplines. Neither does it justify the production of medical graduates who have been instructed rather than educated.

HOW SHOULD CLINICAL STUDENTS OCCUPY THEIR TIME?

Students occupy their time in talking to or examining patients, in being talked to by consultants about patients in the out-patient department or on ward rounds, in listening to lectures (clinical or otherwise), in discussion groups, in studying haematology, microbiology, chemical pathology and morbid histology in the laboratory, in watching postmortem examinations, in watching operations, in talking among themselves and in reading.

Most of this activity usually takes place in their own medical schools or hospitals, though they may make visits to other special hospitals (such as infectious disease or mental hospitals). They may also spend a short period accompanying a GP in his surgery or on his rounds. And they usually spend an elective period of 2 months, which may be at the one extreme in a remote hospital in some distant Third World country or at the other extreme in a district general hospital close to their homes.

A common criticism of the clinical course is that students spend little or no time in general practice, yet in Britain around half of all students are destined to become GPs. In many British medical schools there are departments of General Practice, which no doubt help to redress the balance. On the other hand, these departments can hardly reflect the situation in the ordinary general practice. There is a world of difference between the general practice of prosperous suburbs, of sparsely populated country districts, and of deprived city centres.

There seem to be good reasons why all students should spend a considerable period, say 3 months, towards the end of their clinical course in actually observing general practice. The simplest means of organizing this experience would be to invite GPs who are interested to write to medical schools. They and their practice arrangements could then be vetted by the medical school dean. If deemed satisfactory they could be placed on a list and students would be allotted to them. They would also receive some payment. The value of the scheme could be assessed by obtaining reports both from the students and from the GPs.

Another widespread and justified criticism of medical education is that students spend much of their time in studying rarities. Medical schools collect patients with syringomyelia, motor neurone disease, Addison's disease, various kinds of congenital heart disease, Cushing's syndrome, acromegaly, myasthenia gravis etc. who appear at demonstrations and are repeatedly examined by an endless succession of students. Yet in a lifetime of general practice, very few patients with any of these conditions will be seen. Indeed, a good method of denoting the incidence of maladies is the frequency with which the average GP will see a new case. Looked at this way conditions which in hospitals are common become quite rare. Fry (1978)[6] noted the annual prevalence of illness and other events in the experience of a primary physician caring for a population of 2500 in a developed society. Among them were: one suicide every 4 years, two new carcinomas of the lung and one carcinoma of the breast every year, one new carcinoma of the uterine body every 12 years, one new case of congenital heart disease every 5 years, one new case of Down's syndrome every 10 years, one new case of phenylketonuria every 200 years, and less than one new case of renal failure every year.

Students and their teachers also get a false impression of various common but variable maladies because only the most severe cases gravitate to the hospitals. Some subjects of multiple sclerosis have minimal disability and a life-long remission; many people have minor symptoms from peptic ulcer and remissions lasting years; old people develop advanced osteo-arthropathy but may never complain of it to their doctors; many people have minor rheumatoid arthritis only affecting one or two joints. None of these people are seen in hospital except when they are attending on account of something else. This provides another reason why students should spend some time in general practice.

The situation when the doctor's judgement can be of vital importance, and can sometimes determine whether a patient lives or dies, is when an acute illness develops. The most ill of such patients are usually admitted to hospital. The more of such patients that are seen by the budding GP the better, and he will do this, not by accompanying a GP but by being in a hospital to which emergencies are admitted. Unfortunately, this hospital is too often not the teaching hospital, which is so full up with rare patients having sophisticated investigations that there are no vacancies for emergencies. Indeed, GPs often do not ring up teaching hospitals when they have emergencies, as they know from bitter experience that they will probably be told, perhaps after hanging onto the telephone for 10 minutes, that there is no room. It is true that some teaching hospitals, after pressure from the DHSS, have announced that they are acting as District General Hospitals to the region around them. What a reflection this is on the previous policy of not taking care of the acutely sick who lived in the vicinity!

In my student days some surgical emergencies were admitted to my teaching hospital, but the situation in the medical wards was very different. Emergencies there were a rarity and the beds were almost entirely filled by people who had been seen previously in the out-patient department, or privately in the Harley Street area, and had been put on a waiting list, usually for admission for investigations. Even when medical emergencies were actually brought by ambulance to the hospital they were usually sent on to an LCC hospital. Indeed, virtually none of the patients in the medical wards need have been admitted at all. No doubt the situation is not so bad now as it was then. Nevertheless, many recent students in medical schools where there is both the old teaching hospital and a district general hospital have told me that they have learnt vastly more in the district hospital than in the teaching hospital.

In teaching hospitals there is an enormous emphasis not only on rare syndromes but also on physical signs. Nearly all the 'cases' who attend the examination halls where students have their clinical examinations are chronic subjects with unvarying physical signs. There, students will meet Argyll — Robertson pupils, absent knee jerks, various cardiac murmurs, absent femoral pulses, enlarged spleens, livers and kidneys, Horner's syndrome etc. On their ability to identify these signs may depend whether they pass or fail their exam. Yet in future they will rarely see these signs again. And if they miss or misinterpret one this will probably do no harm. Whereas, if they see a patient with an 'acute abdomen' and decide that there is no need for admission, they may be responsible for his death.

In dealing with acutely ill people the physical signs, or the results of immediate investigations, may greatly influence the action taken. In dealing with chronically unwell the history is often of supreme importance. A large proportion of chronic complainers have no physical signs, and if they do have such signs, they are often irrelevant.

The acutely sick patient usually provides a more testing problem than does the chronic complainer. But the acutely sick cannot be used as examination material for students, so in practice we have to fall back onto the chronic patient. No doubt examiners would claim that physical signs do at least provide objective criteria to aid assessment, whereas for obvious reasons it is difficult to decide whether or not the student has taken a 'correct' history. Moreover, when a patient is telling his history over and over again to a succession of students the whole procedure becomes quite artificial. In the light of all this one may doubt whether a clinical examination, composed as it largely is of chronic patients with physical signs, is a worthwhile test. Certainly, these considerations do not justify the enormous importance which is placed on physical signs both in teaching and examining medical students.

Although students often spend too long a time among the wrong kinds of patients, without doubt the most important activity of the clinical student is to talk to and examine patients. He should also, like other students, engage in a continuous process of discussion with his fellow students and teachers. In this way, it can be hoped, he will be educated rather than instructed.

We often read complaints by medical journalists who are writing about a particular malady that doctors treat the victims of this malady badly because they have been taught so little about it. Alcoholism is one of the commonest 'diseases', we are told, yet medical students spend a few hours throughout their entire course in learning about it. There are innumerable victims of migraine, which journalists typically imply is always a 'torturing pain', and yet students may perhaps not even hear a single lecture wholly devoted to it. Backache is responsible for an enormous amount of absence from work, yet doctors learn little about it and treat its victims abominably (so they go to osteopaths who 'cure' them by manipulation). Medicine is a male-dominated profession, so women's complaints, such as premenstrual tension, are largely ignored, even by women doctors. And so on.

Without doubt students should spend more time looking at patients with common conditions, and especially at patients with acute disasters for whom correct diagnosis is important, and less time on rarities (as I have already noted). But the journalists' belief that by studying a disease one can treat better those affected by it is largely false. When there is some successful treatment we all know about it. Students do not need to spend long hours studying pernicious anaemia to be able to treat those affected by it. We all know that attacks of migraine are said to be sometimes cut short by ergotamine tartrate and to be lessened in severity and frequency by regularly taking clonidine. And we all know that various precipitating factors, such as the menstrual cycle, certain foods, and emotional 'stress', may apparently bring on attacks. But we also know that many patients who have tried these treatments and tried to avoid these factors still complain of attacks. The spending of long hours studying migraine is of little help. The treatment of alcoholism or most kinds of backache is unsatisfactory for the simple reason that there is no satisfactory treatment, however knowledgeable is the doctor. If there were an effective and harmless remedy for premenstrual tension doctors would be delighted to use it but as there is not, no prolonged study of the problem, or getting rid of the alleged male domination of medicine, would make much difference.

Students spend periods attending the specialized departments in the hospital, including geriatric, paediatric, obstetric and gynaecological, psychiatric, eye, ear, nose, and throat, orthopaedic, neurology, rheumatology, and thoracic surgery. Undoubtedly, they can learn much useful information from so doing, provided that the course they are given is tailored to their requirements. But they should also learn much about psychiatry from all their clinical teachers, as psychological aspects are always relevant, especially when dealing with chronic complainers. The predominant trouble of perhaps one third of patients referred to physicians is emotional and much the same is true of those referred to gynaecologists and orthopaedic surgeons. Regrettably, too many consultants fail the students here and even those who readily admit the importance of the psyche may nevertheless take the attitude that their concern is to deal with organic disease or to demonstrate that no such disease is present.

Although so many patients in hospital are elderly, most of them are in the general wards, with an especially high proportion in the medical, orthopaedic, and ophthalmic wards. In most hospitals the geriatric wards are largely filled with longterm occupants, the majority of whom remain there until they die. Even if students never go to the geriatric wards, they can hardly be unaware of the high incidence of most illness among the old. No doubt students should spend some time in the geriatric wards, and if for a spell they act as orderlies they can gain a worthwhile understanding of the practical problems of looking after the aged chronic sick. But there are no great principles to be learned in the geriatric wards. And the idea that a particular expertise is needed to treat the maladies of the old is largely false (see Chapter 7).

On the other hand, students should spend considerable time among children and in particular in seeing acutely sick children. Although the vast majority of acute illnesses in children are self-limiting, for a few, such as acute appendicitis, meningitis, or intussusception, treatment can be life-saving. The GP's decision whether or not to admit a child with one of these conditions can determine whether he lives or dies. It matters little whether or not students see examples of the rarities which tend to gravitate to children's hospitals.

Students should also see as many as possible of orthopaedic and rheumatic patients and gynaecological patients, since these provide so many of the problems of general practice. Moreover, such patients usually provide a general rather than a specialist problem. They will therefore fare much better under the care of a GP who looks at them as people than under the care of an orthopaedic surgeon who confines his attention to the region of which they complain or of the gynaecologist who may shut his eyes to everything except what is visible through a vaginal speculum.

Accepting that the supremely important element of the clinical student's life is to be involved with patients, is it possible to reach any valid conclusions as to how much time should be devoted to private reading, formal lectures, attending the pathological laboratory, looking at operations and other activities? In any case, whatever conclusions are reached, to a considerable extent the student himself decides how he should spend his time. Some students spend long hours in reading, making copious notes as they do so, whereas others read very little. Some students work hard, whereas others appear bone-idle and spend long hours in the common-room.

Reading is potentially of enormous value. On the other hand, just as some teachers instruct rather than educate students, so may some students amass information from reading without acquiring any general understanding of a problem. In my student days many of the well known textbooks were appallingly bad in that their authors were totally uncritical. In particular, long lists of recommended treatments were laid down to be 'essential' and various activities were 'forbidden', although there was absolutely no evidence that the treatments were beneficial or the activities harmful. Today's textbooks are no doubt better than yesterday's, but treatments of unproven value are still recommended for theoretical reasons and dubious statements about aetiology are still made. We may read that various maladies can be brought on by 'stress', without it being made clear that 'stress' cannot be measured or even satisfactorily defined. We are sometimes informed that 'it is generally thought that' or 'most physicians believe that', as if consensus proves anything. We all agree that in the past most physicians believed all sorts of grotesque absurdities.

Courses of formal lectures have often been derided on the ground that they are essentially the same as textbooks yet have the serious disadvantage that the lecturer goes at his own pace, whereas when a student reads a textbook he can take the difficult passages slowly and re-read them until he is sure he understands what has been written. In the mediaeval universities before the invention of printing the only way the student could learn the message of some Master was to trudge across Europe to the Master's university and sit at his feet. The modern student merely needs to buy the Master's book. Perhaps courses of formal lectures are merely a carry over from those remote days. On the other hand, an inspiring lecturer can get his message across in a way that a book cannot. And some students insist that they can remember what they are taught in lectures whereas they forget what they have learnt in books. When lectures are illustrated by slides or are accompanied by demonstrations they may of course provide something beyond the scope of any book. In general, much better than formal lectures are tutorials or discussion groups in which the students can ask questions and advance their views.

In my student days students spent long hours in operating theatres. Some surgeons had very long lists, and I well remember staying from 2 pm until 8 pm or even later, and of being filled with justifiable pride as a result. But most of the time one could see little or nothing of what was going on, and in so far as one could see, very little of value was learnt. This time spent in operating theatres was largely wasted. Today's students do not spend such long hours in this largely futile activity. It seems reasonable that a student should be scrubbed up when 'his' patients are being operated on, as he is then actually taking part by holding a retractor or other instrument.

He also learns in a practical way about surgical technique and he can see what is happening. But otherwise it seems doubtful whether students should go to operating theatres.

VALUE OF AND COST OF INVESTIGATIONS

A striking feature of the medical scene throughout the affluent world is the investigation explosion.

Unfortunately, whereas present day clinical teachers are more critical of treatment than were their predecessors, there is little sign that many are critical of the value of investigations. Too often it is just taken for granted that it is a Good Thing to do an enormous series of investigations. Many clinicians, physicians especially, lay down that certain investigations should be done as routine. Some physicians will hardly look at a patient until he has had a large number of investigations. And in teaching hospitals many more investigations tend to be done than in other hospitals, partly because there is more sophisticated equipment to carry them out. All this is considered in Chapter 5. In my resident days in my teaching hospital I recall asking physicians why certain investigations were done, since the diagnosis was already clear. The physicians agreed that the investigations were superfluous, but they were done *for the sake of the students.* How remarkable it was that students should be deliberately given the impression that unnecessary investigations should be done! Present-day medical students have told me that this same excuse for doing investigations is still made.

Here, the age old question posed by Juvenal, *'quis custodiet ipsos custodes?'* becomes particularly apt. If the eminent physicians in the teaching hospitals themselves use investigations with so total a lack of discrimination, how can students be expected to do better when they go out into the world?

A glimmer of hope in this depressing situation is to be seen in the recent suggestion of some disenchantment with High Technology. Many people, even in the United States, are asking whether the practice of doing numerous investigations on uncomplaining people does more harm than good, as well as being wasteful. Elaborate machines are perhaps not worshipped to the extent that they were a few years ago.

THE COST OF TREATMENT

Doctors are commonly accused of having little concept of the enormous cost of treatment. In particular, they are said to be unaware of the extreme differences in the cost of drugs, in spite of the regular bulletins on this matter which are sent to all doctors by the DHSS. No doubt these bulletins frequently go straight into the waste-paper basket. Expensive drugs continue to be prescribed in circumstances when cheaper ones would do just as well. Most students are told little about the cost of treatment.

It can be argued that the brains of medical students are already stuffed too full of facts, and that to expect them also to know the cost of treatment is unreasonable. Certainly, if during their course students were given formal lectures on this matter, one could hardly expect them to be interested or to remember much of what they were told. But if clinicians, pharmacologists, and pharmacists regularly mentioned the cost when they were talking to students about treatment, this would be likely to have a much greater impact. Especial emphasis should be placed on the most expensive kinds of treatment such as blood transfusion. When a patient was thought to need a transfusion in my resident days, I personally would get in touch with the relatives or with the patient's place of work and ask for volunteers. I would then group, cross-match, and bleed them. All this was an effective deterrent to giving transfusions without good cause. The modern resident merely has to sign a form to say 'Cross match six units' and then do no more than insert a cannula into a vein. The great number of man-hours, the complex organization, and the vast cost of producing those six units of blood are easily overlooked. Once more, the deficiencies in the students' education are due to the deficiencies in the teachers, who too often fail even to mention the cost of treatment.

SUMMARY

(1) A broad education before medical school is intrinsically

desirable. This produces better citizens, though there is no clear evidence that it produces better doctors.

(2) The most important pre-clinical subjects are chemistry and physiology (including biochemistry and pharmacology). Physics and anatomy are less important. A knowledge of biology should be part of every liberal education.

(3) Medical students have been too often instructed rather than educated. Rather than being encouraged to think for themselves and to criticize, they have been force-fed with information and been the recipients of *ex cathedra* pronouncements from consultants. This approach has been defended on the grounds that medicine is an art as well as a science. The belief that the practice of medicine involves the two antithetical approaches of art and science is false.

(4) Clinical students should all spend a period attached to a general practitioner. Far to great an emphasis is placed on rarities and especially chronic rarities, both in teaching and in examinations. Students should spend much of their time among patients, with especial emphasis on acute emergencies (who are seen so rarely in many teaching hospitals).

(5) Students should learn about the psychological aspects of maladies, not just from psychiatrists, but from all clinicians. Many clinicians fail to give this teaching.

(6) Courses of formal lectures are of doubtful value. Apart from direct involvement with patients, students should spend most of their time in reading, discussion, tutorials, and in the pathological laboratory. They should spend little time in operating theatres.

(7) Students should be made aware of the value and cost of investigations. Too often, their teachers overvalue investigations. Students should also learn about the cost of treatment, not as a separate subject, but regularly whenever treatment is prescribed.

References

1. Pickering, G.W. (1958). *Br. Med. J.*, **2**, 1117
2. Porritt, A.E. (1960). *Br. Med. J.*, **1**, 1907

3. Lawrence, R.D. (1950). *Br. Med. J.*, **2**, 481
4. Annotation (1959). *Practitioner*, **182**, 143
5. Collier, H.E. (1950). *Med. World*, **72**, 867
6. Fry, J. (1978). *A New Approach to Medicine* (Lancaster: MTP Press)

2

The Nature of Maladies

Medical students are given the impression that patients are affected by a disease. And a disease is thought to have an independent reality. As Pickering (1962) says[1], 'We have grown accustomed to defining a disease, and ultimately to ascribing it, to a unique and specific fault with a unique and specific cause'. Although we all realize how difficult it can be to reach a diagnosis, we may still take it for granted that, if only we were more knowledgeable and more clever, we could still attach some neat diagnostic label to every patient. When faced by a patient who has defied all the efforts of mortal man, we may perhaps assume that the Almighty would know which particular disease was responsible for the illness.

There is also an endless debate as to whether some malady is a disease, or a disease 'in its own right', or a disease *sui generis*, or an entity, or whether it is merely a syndrome or two or three or any number of different entities. Thus: 'Diabetes mellitus is now accepted to be a syndrome rather than a single disease' (Bottazo and others, 1978)[2]; 'Its many modes of presentation and its various patterns of progress make one wonder if (rheumatoid arthritis) is not several pathological processes with many different starting factors rather than a single entity' (Hart, 1972)[3]; 'Polymyalgia rheumatica is a distinct clinical entity' (Huskisson, and others, 1977)[4]. 'Another set of results implying that schizophrenia is a

21

specific biochemical entity was reported by Bird' (*British Medical Journal*, leading article, 1977)[5].

How, then, can a disease or an entity be defined? According to the *Shorter Oxford Dictionary* a disease is 'A condition of the body ... in which its functions are disturbed and or deranged, illness, sickness; an ailment' and an entity is 'Being; existence ... that which makes a thing what it is; essence ... an ENS, as distinct from a function, attribute, relation etc .... Being generally'.

These complicated definitions give us no help in understanding the nature of patients' illnesses. In practice, some maladies are clear-cut and can reasonably be described as diseases or entities. This is true of specific infections. A patient with a lung which has being partially destroyed by the *M. tuberculosis* is suffering from the disease tuberculosis and the patient with dementia due to *Treponema pallidum* in his brain has the disease syphilis. Non-specific infections such as boils or whitlows are also entities. The same is true of malignant conditions. As a rule the firm conclusion can be reached, either clinically or by biopsy, that a woman has, or has not, the entity carcinoma of the breast. There are, it is true, conditions in the uncertain territory between the benign and the malignant. Is carcinoma *in situ* of the cervix uteri the same entity as invasive carcinoma? Although this question cannot easily be answered, this does not affect the general conclusion that we can usually decide with confidence whether or not a patient has a carcinoma. Myocardial infarct and cerebral infarct are entities. Here the problem may arise of deciding whether or not a patient has suffered one of them. For it is impossible to prove that someone has not had a minor cardiac or cerebral infarct (though the absurd claim used to be made by eminent cardiologists that a repeatedly normal twelve lead e.c.g. proved that a patient had not had a cardiac infarct).

But when we consider many other maladies the situation is quite different. We are told that there are over 200 distinct rheumatic conditions and those who say this evidently believe that all these are in some sense separate entities. Rheumatoid arthritis is usually thought to be one entity, ankylosing spondylitis a second, psoriatic arthropathy a third, colitic arthropathy a fourth, Reiter's disease a fifth, 'polymyalgia rheumatica' a sixth, osteoarthropathy a seventh, and so on indefinitely.

Some rheumatic conditions can be clearly separated from the others. Gout is associated with a disturbance of uric acid metabolism and the clinical picture is usually characteristic. Rheumatic fever can be precisely defined, because of its relation to beta haemolytic streptococcal infection. And the classical case of rheumatic fever can be confused with nothing else. But even here there can be difficulties. What label should be given to a child who has had a streptococcal throat infection and 2 weeks later develops some minor limb pains for a day or two, without fever or malaise? About half the victims of rheumatic heart disease give no history suggesting rheumatic fever. Should we conclude that they *must* have had subclinical rheumatic fever? No satisfactory answer can be given to such questions.

Patients who are given the diagnosis of rheumatoid arthritis vary enormously. At the one extreme is the patient with minor affection of one or two metacarpo-phalangeal joints whilst at the other extreme is the bedridden patient with ankylosis of nearly every joint. As noted above, Hart wondered if rheumatoid arthritis is not several pathological processes rather than a single entity. One might lay down an arbitrary definition that single joint disease is one entity, two joint disease a second, three joint disease a third, and so on. But this seems wholly futile. A patient with ankylosing spondylitis may have, in addition to his spinal troubles, affection of the large limb joints which appears just the same as that of rheumatoid arthritis. Yet rheumatoid arthritis and ankylosing spondylitis are said, at least in Europe, to be separate entities. 'Polymyalgia rheumatica' has in recent years become a popular label, and is given to patients, mostly elderly, with widespread pain, especially across the shoulder girdle, without evidence of joint disease and accompanied by a high ESR and constitutional symptoms such as sweating, low fever, weight loss and depression, responding dramatically to a small dose of steroid. But if a patient has a high ESR and constitutional disturbance, responds to steroid but never complains of pain (and is not in fact suffering from occult malignant disease) is he affected by 'polymyalgia rheumatica'? A diagnosis which implies - as does 'polymyalgia rheumatica' - that a patient must have pain is unsatisfactory.

The best way of dealing with the rheumatic conditions is to get away from the concept of separate disease entities. The statement that there are over 200, or 100, or 300, or any other figure, distinct rheumatic conditions is both meaningless and valueless. Rather should we view the rheumatic diseases as an ill-defined group of maladies affecting the joints and soft tissues, and often associated with disorders of other organs, which are infinitely variable in symptomatology and severity. Reaching this conclusion does not imply that all the old familiar labels such as rheumatoid arthritis, colitic arthropathy, Reiter's disease etc. are worthless. On the contrary, such labels may be helpful. We should merely rid ourselves of the idea that they have a precise meaning and are, in Pickering's words, 'a unique and specific fault with a unique and specific cause'.

Any number of other examples which illustrate this problem can be given. Are epilepsy, essential hypertension, and the 'irritable bowel syndrome' diseases or entities? Epilepsy which is related to brain disease is clearly distinct from epilepsy which is thought to be idiopathic. But idiopathic epilepsy varies infinitely. Do patients with grand mal, petit mal, and psychomotor attacks have the same entity? The blood pressure is infinitely variable. Above what level should the term essential hypertension be used? And is this an entity? The 'irritable bowel syndrome' is a convenient label to apply to nervous and introspective subjects with abdominal discomfort and variable motions. Is it a disease?

If the concept of separate disease entities is unsatisfactory when dealing with the maladies of the body, it can be doubly unsatisfactory in dealing with the disorders of the mind. We can distinguish between mental disorder associated with brain disease and mental disorder which is thought to be solely 'in the mind'. Organically caused mental disorder is generally thought to be more 'real' than such disorder 'in the mind'. There is in consequence a desire to hypothesize organic brain changes to explain mental disorder. In particular, schizophrenia is thought by many to be really a brain disease or a 'specific biochemical entity' (see p. 22 above), although it is placed among the mental disorders in the conventional textbooks. Perhaps there is a common assumption that the psychoses are 'really' organic, whereas the neuroses are just in the mind. But it is absurd to consider such labels as anxiety state, involutional melancholia, endogenous depression, hysteria and psychopathic personality as separate entities. For there is every gradation ranging from the balanced individual through minor states of anxiety and depression to advanced schizophrenia or profound melancholia.

When medical writers are considering specific infections or neoplasms they do not refer to them as entities. No-one solemnly states: 'Carcinoma of the breast is an entity'. In practice we only read of entities, or diseases in their own right, or diseases *sui generis* when the rheumatic disorders or schizophrenia or other indefinite conditions are under review.

It may be argued that, although in the light of present knowledge the view I am advancing is sound, if only our knowledge could be more advanced we should be able to define many more entities. In the mid 19th century many of the illnesses accompanied by fever could hardly be distinguished. We then had short fever, recurrent fever, low fever, and continued fever, whereas now we can distinguish typhoid, paratyphoid, typhus, tuberculosis and so on. There may well be some truth in this, and in 20 years we shall no doubt be aware of more entities than we are now. But there seems no ground for supposing that we shall ever be able to separate the rheumatic maladies and many others into clear-cut entities. Any attempt to classify the mental disorders into entities will always be absurd. Entities and diseases are devised by us to enable us to understand our patients better; there is no reason to believe that they are or ever will be a reflection of eternal Truth.

The desire to discover 'real' diseases has had the unfortunate effect of encouraging doctors to hypothesize pathological states which have no reality, or of wrongly associating the patient's symptoms with some incidental abnormality. During the First World War vast numbers of soldiers were given the diagnoses of shell-shock and 'disordered action of the heart'. Shell-shock was supposed to be a disease of the central nervous system caused by proximity to explosions and disordered action of the heart was thought to be a cardiac disease. In fact, the symptoms of both groups were the somatic manifestations of emotional disorder, which was obvious if the soldiers were looked at as whole men, not as conglomerations of organs (see also Chapter 3, p. 38) Between the wars the various ptoses explained the abdominal symptoms of innumerable chronic complainers. Until recent years among the commonest of all diagnoses were 'fibrositis' and 'neuritis', which explained much pain in the limbs and back and which were described in the text-book with full pathological details. (See Chapter 8, p. 136).

Perhaps we are now more humble than were our predecessors, who, we are told, would lay down dogmatically that the diagnosis was so and so. There is now a widespread realization that so many maladies are not satisfactorily explained. Numerous patients whom in the past would have been given an organic diagnosis would now be deemed, except by the most mechanistically inclined, to have the somatic manifestations of emotional disorder. The severity of all symptoms with an evident organic cause is determined both by the state of the body and the state of the mind. But even if we consider only patients with organic maladies, a large proportion cannot be given a clear-cut pathological diagnosis. This is especially true of those who complain of headache, backache, and bellyache, which are the commonest somatic symptoms.

HEADACHE

Much headache and other head sensations are evidently related to the emotional state. The head sensations of which depressed, tense and worried people complain tend to be widespread and persistent. The patient may insist that they are continuous for days, months, or even years at a time. They are typically described as like a tight band, like a feeling of pressure, or bursting and are unrelieved by analgesics.

A tiny proportion of headache is due to some gross organic disease, such as meningitis, subarachnoid haemorrhage, cranial arteritis, or cerebral tumour. As a rule the other manifestations make the diagnosis apparent, except sometimes when the headache is due to a slowly growing cerebral tumour.

In the past, and to some extent now, much headache has been wrongly attributed to various organic conditions. One popular explanation used to be an error of refraction, and many headache sufferers used to be (and some still are) referred for sight testing, commonly departing with a prescription for spectacles. It was even claimed that minor degrees of astigmatism caused headache whereas major degrees did not. There may well be a few people with severe errors of refraction who need, but do not wear, spectacles and consequently suffer headache. But, leaving them aside, there appears no good evidence that refractive errors are responsible for headache.

When headache is associated with hypertension the error may be made of assuming that the headache is caused by hypertension. Indeed, when patients are told they have a raised blood pressure they may begin to complain of headache (of which they were previously free). Malignant hypertension with papilloedema does result in headache, but otherwise there appear to be no good grounds for hypothesizing ' hypertensive headache '. And, remarkably, even some patients with the full-blown picture of ' malignant hypertension ' do not complain of headache.

Headache is often attributed to sinusitis. Patients who, perhaps many years before, were told that their headaches were due to sinus may for ever after take it for granted that whenever they get a headache ' sinus ' is responsible. They may indeed refer to ' my sinus headaches '. Acute infection in the sinuses may undoubtedly be associated with pain. Frontal sinusitis may result in pain and localized tenderness in the forehead. Suppuration in the antra may be accompanied by pain or discomfort in the face. But in these situations there is overt evidence of acute infection in the sinuses.

The practical question is: 'Is headache ever caused by sinusitis in the absence of obvious clinical evidence of sinusitis?'. When patients with headache are investigated, abnormalities in the sinuses may be found. X-rays may reveal opacity or what is thought to be ' thickened lining membrane '. Occasionally antral puncture may reveal pus. But there appears to be no good evidence that frontal, vertical, occipital or widespread headache can be related to such abnormalities in the sinuses.

Much headache has been attributed to various ' rheumatic ' conditions, including cervical spondylopathy, "fibrositis" or ' myalgia ' of the scalp, and ' neuralgia '. Cervical spondylopathy can undoubtedly cause pain in the neck and down the arms and perhaps in the head. But here there is overt evidence of a painful neck. Headache is sometimes attributed to spondylopathy solely on account of X-ray changes in the neck but this has no justification. ' Fibrositis ' has been largely debunked. Patients who complain of recurrent stabbing head pains may be said to have neuralgia and they may make this diagnosis themselves. The symptoms of many of the patients who have been said to have 'rheumatic' headache appear to be largely or wholly psychogenic.

Most recurrent headache is in practice said to be migraine, and this is generally thought to be due to spasm, followed by dilatation, of some cerebral vessels (though this belief has been questioned). The "classical" migraine subject has recurrent attacks beginning with visual symptoms and followed by headache, often unilateral, and sometimes vomiting. If a patient merely complains of recurrent headache alone, should that be described as migraine? No satisfactory answer can be given to this question.

Migraine is organic in the sense that it is thought to be related to temporary disturbance of the cerebral vessels, but it is not organic in the more usual sense of implying a gross lesion. It can be put under the category of 'functional' disorders, when ' functional ' is used, not as an alternative to neurotic or psychogenic, as it so often is, but to indicate a temporary disturbance of bodily function. (See Chapter 3, p. 43).

Unless it can be called migraine, most recurrent headache cannot be related even to a transient pathological process. Some of it is psychogenic but much of it is not. However, even when headache has no known pathological basis, its cause in the aetiological sense may be obvious. This is true of the headache which follows an alcoholic carouse, exposure to a hot sun, or associated with a loaded rectum. Even when headache follows minor trauma, we do not understand the precise mechanism of the headache, although it is evidently related to damage to some of the coverings of the brain.

BACKACHE

Like headache, much backache reflects the patient's emotional state. Those who are tired and depressed often complain of low backache. When this is persistent for long periods, little affected by posture, little relieved by analgesics, and is associated with various other symptoms, the backache is likely to be largely or wholly psychogenic. Perhaps the archetypal patient with predominantly psychogenic backache is the overweight, depressed, middle-aged woman who spends a boring life doing her endless domestic chores.

There is a particular psychological aspect of backache which is less often related to other chronic pains - the compensation problem. Damage to the back is common in industrial and road accidents, and backache is a regular sequel of such accidents. The greater and more prolonged the pain, the larger is the monetary compensation likely to be, so there is a strong temptation to exaggerate the pain. Features which suggest that the pain is being exaggerated are its description in extravagant terms, its bizarre distribution, and the failure to respond to analgesics. During the war it was widely believed by service medical officers that the complaint of non-existent backache was the commonest form of malingering. And, although the usual reason for this was to escape from the horrors of battle, it was often said that the prospect of a long route march might cause some soldiers to report sick with 'backache', especially if there was a green young medical officer.

A small proportion of backache is caused by gross diseases such as metastases in the spine, spinal cord tumours, and ankylosing spondylitis. But the vast majority of backache which appears to be due to some organic process has no such obvious cause. It may be impossible to reach any firm pathological diagnosis. Unfortunately, doctors have habitually made unjustified pathological diagnoses to explain backache (See also Chapter 8). Before the war common backache diagnoses were fibrositis, neuritis, sacroiliac strain, sacroiliac arthritis, lumbo-sacral back strain, and retroverted uterus (which was said to be the commonest cause of low backache in women, and operations were done for its correction). Criteria were laid down in the textbooks to distinguish between these conditions. The "neuritis" which was the supposed cause of most sciatica was discussed with full pathological details (and the patient was treated by painting iodine along the course of the nerve, thus giving relief by the mechanism of counter-irritation).

These particular diagnoses have largely died out. But there remains a tendency to attribute backache to some radiological or other abnormality which in fact is coincidental. When a middle-age backache victim is X-rayed he may be found to have calcified spurs on some of his vertebrae. These spurs have probably no connection with the backache, but the patient may be informed that he has 'arthritis of the spine', and thereafter take it for granted that this is the cause of his backache. The spine X-rays of old people frequently show wedging of one or more vertebrae resulting from crush fractures in the past. This may sometimes be related to backache, but the same appearances are common in those who do not complain of their backs. And there are no clear criteria to distinguish between those with backache due to the wedging and those with backache due to something else.

The pathological process underlying backache which now looms so large is the damaged intervertebral disc. Knowledgeable patients may complain, not of backache but of 'slipped disc', and they explain the coming and going of their ache by the slipping in and out of their discs. Without doubt, much low back and leg pain is related to pressure on nerves from a protruded disc. Are there clear criteria which distinguish backache due to a disc lesion and backache due to other causes?

A few years ago it was widely believed that when backache is accompanied by sciatic or femoral nerve pain and especially when there is objective evidence of nerve involvement (such as blunting of knee or ankle jerks or wasting of calf muscles or quadriceps) this was virtually diagnostic of prolapsed disc. No doubt many patients with this picture have disc lesions, but others do not, as laminectomy may fail to reveal a prolapsed disc. Other diagnoses have recently become popular. Lumbar spinal stenosis, either apparently idiopathic or due to a variety of pathological processes other than prolapsed disc, is thought by some to be an important cause of low back and leg pain. ' Lumbar instability ' is also said to be an important cause of backache. This has been defined as "a loss of integrity of soft-tissue intersegmental control, causing potential weakness and liability to yield under stress' (Newman, 1973)[6]. It has been said to be one of the commonest causes of back pain. Spinous process impingement provides one more explanation of backache.

In practice it is, therefore, often impossible to make a firm pathological diagnosis of back pain. It is a universal complaint which usually clears up in due course. Nevertheless, as with headache, the cause in the aetiological sense may be clear, although the mechanism by which this is responsible for pain remains obscure. Any strenuous activity involving the back may evidently be responsible for subsequent backache. This typically happens to the weekend gardener. During the week his back rarely troubles him, but after spending a day in weeding and digging he may later have widespread backache and be unable to straighten his back without discomfort. Those who drive cars for long periods are liable to backache which is evidently due to their posture while driving. In the older textbooks backache was sometimes attributed to ' faulty posture', 'chronic fatigue', or 'inadequate' rest. Such theories cannot be proved, but they illustrate that backache may be thought to have a cause in the aetiological sense without a cause in the pathological sense.

Among the health-conscious public there is a common belief that doctors are not much use in dealing with backache. This is of course true in the sense that the course of events is usually uninfluenced by anything done by doctors (apart from prescribing analgesics). Cults have developed, the followers of which claim to have particular expertise in dealing with the back. The best known is osteopathy, which is considered in Chapter 9, p. 177.

BELLYACHE

Whereas most headache and backache cannot be related to any known pathological process, much bellyache can be so explained. Probably the commonest cause of bellyache is acute "gastro-enteritis" due to organisms or chemical irritants. Other familiar causes of bellyache are peptic ulcer, cholecystitis, pancreatitis, diverticulitis, acute or recurrent appendicitis and colitis.

A good deal of bellyache is nevertheless unexplained pathologically. This is especially true of long-standing and persistent bellyache. Here, the symptoms are often largely or wholly of emotional origin. The features which suggest an emotional basis is that the ache is persistent, perhaps for months on end, often widespread, unrelated to meals, imperfectly relieved or unrelieved by drugs, and described in exaggerated terms. There are typically associated bodily symptoms, such as ' wind ', constipation, exhaustion, tiredness and general malaise, and there may be overt evidence of depression or anxiety.

Even more than with headache and backache there has been a common tendency to hypothesize various pathological states to explain bellyache, or to relate it to various abnormalities which happen to be present. In my student days a familiar *ex cathedra* pronouncement made by surgeons was: 'The commonest cause of abdominal pain is constipation'. Even if this were true, it would demand the further question: 'What is the cause of the constipation?'. Patients, usually elderly, are seen who have had no proper bowel motion for a long time and complain of abdominal and rectal discomfort and are found to have a mass of impacted faeces (and their symptoms are promptly relieved when the bowel is emptied by an enema). But apart from this situation, there appear to be no good grounds for attributing persistent bellyache to constipation. This is in any case impossible to define and the diagnosis of constipation is usually made by the patient, who believes that his motions are less frequent than they should be. On the other hand, certain symptoms are undoubtedly related to constipation. When a patient has an anal fissure the act of defaecation can be so painful that the desire to stool is suppressed, so the fissure is the cause of constipation. And the passage of a hard faecal mass, which can reasonably be considered a feature of constipation, is more or less painful and may cause rectal damage.

Persistent or frequently recurring pain in the right iliac fossa, perhaps accompanied by such other symptoms as nausea, anorexia and malaise, used to be attributed to 'chronic appendicitis'. The diagnosis was confirmed by finding persistent tenderness over McBurney's point or by demonstration of a kinked, fixed and non-filling appendix by barium enema X-ray. And surgeons claimed that patients with such symptoms were cured by the removal of their appendixes, even when these looked normal. Such claims were anecdotal and there is no convincing evidence that appendicectomy in such patients as these is in the long run beneficial. ''Chronic appendicitis ' has no proven reality. ' Chronic cholecystitis ' also used to be a popular diagnosis and was said to be a common cause of flatulent dyspepsia in fat middle-aged women, usually accompanied by gall-stones. Aching and tenderness in the region of the gall-bladder, a non-secreting or poorly secreting gall-bladder in the cholecystogram and a history of fat intolerance were said to be confirmatory findings. In fact, there appears to be no good evidence that fat intolerance in those with gall-stones is commoner than in those who are free of stones and much of the alleged fat intolerance follows the patient being told that she has stones, as everyone ' knows ' that those with gall-stones should avoid fatty foods. The diagnosis of "chronic cholecystitis" should be just as suspect as that of 'chronic appendicitis'.

Between the wars much abdominal pain was attributed to visceroptosis or to particular ptoses such as gastroptosis or nephroptosis. Consequently, unfortunate patients had operations to cure the ptoses or belts to hold the displaced viscera in place. At the same time upper abdominal pain with other symptoms was attributed to ' gastritis ' (which could be seen through the recently introduced flexible gastroscope). Intestinal auto-intoxication was one more bogus diagnosis. Fortunately, these diagnoses are now almost dead.

Persistent or recurrent pain which appears to arise from the colon is common and may be accompanied by tenderness in either iliac fossa and often by a palpable, as well as tender, descending colon. Such pain may be associated with bowel irregularity and is seen especially in emotionally disturbed women, who usually have various other somatic symptoms. The current popular diagnosis in this situation is the ' irritable bowel syndrome ', which seems a reasonable label, since it does not imply any pathological process and does indicate the nature of the symptoms. In many such patients a psychological diagnosis is appropriate, as the abdominal symptoms evidently reflect an emotional disturbance.

EMOTIONAL ASPECTS OF ORGANIC DISEASE

When a patient has some undoubted organic lesion the mere statement that ' the diagnosis ' is this lesion remains incomplete, for the severity and nature of the symptoms are not wholly determined by the nature of the lesion; they are also determined by the emotional state. In practice, this is relevant to chronic conditions. When a patient has some acute condition, such as acute appendicitis or coronary thrombosis, we know that the complaints of the phlegmatic unimaginitive individual will be very different from those of the nervous and worrying person. The former may merely say that he has developed a pain in his belly or chest, whereas the latter may be in an extreme state of alarm and believe he is about to die. But all this does not much affect the handling of the situation. The surgeon will advise appendicectomy for both the patients with appendicitis, and after the acute episode is over, both will once more become much the same as they had been before. And the physician will manage both coronary patients in much the same way, though the nervous subject will no doubt be more heavily sedated and, it must be hoped, more thoroughly and repeatedly reassured. Here, the end result may be different, as the phlegmatic individual may become symptom-free, whereas the nervous one may have persistent symptoms such as palpitation, exhaustion, and left mammary aching which he believes are due to his damaged heart, but are in fact emotional in origin. Perhaps continued reassurance and encouragement will help to minimize these symptoms.

When patients have progressive chronic diseases, the nature of their complaints may vary greatly, according to their temperaments. A few people can apparently accept with equanimity that they are slowly dying. Here, too, the doctor's handling of the situation will be affected by the emotional aspects, but the important treatment, if such exists, will be the same in both cases.

If the process of making a full diagnosis is to explain the patient's symptoms, the emotional aspects may be supremely important when the organic lesion is chronic but non-fatal. If a man with a sebaceous cyst which he is convinced is a cancer is merely given the diagnosis ' sebaceous cyst ' he is being diagnosed wrongly. Only a doctor with a remarkably narrow and mechanistic outlook could make so gross an error. But when the psychological element is not so conspicuous a purely organic diagnosis which is seriously incomplete can be made more easily. The subject of mitral stenosis with a well-functioning heart may be worried about himself and complain of dizziness, exhaustion and palpitation. The bald diagnosis ' mitral stenosis ' is clearly wrong and the diagnosis should be ' mitral stenosis in a nervous, worrying man with psychosomatic symptoms which he wrongly thinks are due to the diseased state of his heart '. The doctor who makes this correct diagnosis may be able to lessen the patient's symptoms by his reassurance and encouragement.

This kind of diagnostic error may have especially bad effects when operation is under consideration. The surgeon may operate on a woman with varicose veins because of her insistence that her veins are aching. But the surgeon who looks at patients as people, not just at that part of the body of which they complain, can see that this aching is not directly due to the veins; it is due to the patient's consciousness of their existence and of their ugly appearance. Admittedly, if the operation abolishes the varicosities the patient may say that her aching has gone, so the operation was justified. When varicosities in women are gross and ugly operation is indeed justified for cosmetic reasons, but when a woman has small and not very conspicuous varicosities, the surgeon should probably not recommend operation. Instead, he should explain that the aching is not due to the veins and emphasize that the legs do not look ugly. Similarly the nervous and worrying patient who knows she has gall-stones may have a variety of symptoms such as flatulent dyspepsia and fat intolerance. The surgeon who explains that gall-stones do not cause such symptoms and that one woman in five has gall-stones may be able to help the patient without removing her gall-bladder.

THE SINGLE WORD DIAGNOSIS

Although the public expect the doctor to make a single word or single phrase diagnosis, in practice this is only possible with some acute conditions. 'Boil', 'whitlow', 'common cold', 'tonsillitis' and 'carious tooth' are familiar single word or phrase diagnoses which satisfactorily explain the symptoms. But when dealing with many acute or recurrent conditions, including much headache, backache and bellyache and all chronic conditions, the single word diagnosis is inappropriate or absurd. A diagnosis is an explanation of a patient's malady; so often this explanation needs a long sentence.

SUMMARY

(1) Some maladies can rightly be considered as diseases or entities, but many cannot. This is notably true of the rheumatic conditions and psychological disorders.

(2) Because of the desire to discover gross pathological processes, many maladies have wrongly been attributed to such processes, which have either been fanciful or have been associated but irrelevant abnormalities. And in teaching medical students far too much emphasis has been placed on those few patients with gross and ' interesting ' pathological states and exciting physical signs.

(3) Even when somatic symptoms are evidently related to organic processes, it is often impossible to incriminate any particular lesion. This is true of much backache, headache, and bellyache. But we can often determine the aetiology of a malady, although we are ignorant of the pathology.

(4) To diagnose is to explain the patient's symptoms, and even when some organic process is clearly related to the symptoms, their severity and nature are also determined by the state of mind. This is especially relevant to patients with chronic benign lesions.

(5) The single word diagnosis is only appropriate for acute conditions.

References

1. Pickering, G.W. (1962). *Lancet,* 1, 1298
2. Bottazzo, G.E. and others. (1978). *Br. Med. J.,* 2, 253
3. Hart, F.D. (1972). *Br. Med. J.,* 2, 621
4. Huskisson, E.C. and others. (1977). *Br. Med. J.,* 2, 1459
5. Leading article (1977). *Br. Med. J.,* 2, 976
6. Newman, P.H. (1973). *J. Bone J. Surg.,* 55B, 7

3

Psychosomatic and Functional Disorders

Everyone knows that somatic symptoms are often due to psychological causes. The very words of the English language indicate that the heart is the seat of the emotions. People speak of affairs of the heart when they mean affairs of love. A man's heart is said to rule his head when his feelings are stronger than his reason. People are said to be sad at heart when depressed and it is said that their hearts are bitter when angry and that someone who has suffered a tragedy is broken-hearted. We also speak of being sick with grief, speechless with rage and trembling with emotion, and people are said to lose their appetites when crossed in love, to vomit with disgust, to develop diarrhoea from anxiety, to go into a cold sweat from fear, or to blush with shame.

Yet during the Dark Age of medicine in the thirties, when I was educated, nearly all somatic symptoms were explained on an organic basis. Patients were considered to be ' clinical material ' (this awful phrase was often heard) in whom disease had to be identified or excluded. Even those consultants who were kind and polite did not take patients aside and ask them about their personal problems.

The patient who complained of palpitation, dizziness, left mammary aching, sighing respiration, and fatigue was said, at least by many physicians, to have an irritable heart, effort syndrome, or disordered action of the heart. In Price's *Practice of Medicine,* a most popular textbook of the time, there were long sections devoted to ' Primary Cardiac Overstrain ' and ' Soldier's Heart ' (or Disordered Action of the Heart) with exhaustive discussion about aetiology and pathology. Among the symptoms of both diseases were lassitude, languor, palpitation, a feeling of oppression or constriction of the chest, tremors, nervousness, insomnia, vertigo, dull headache, hebetude and fainting attacks i.e. just the symptoms which seem to us obviously of emotional origin.

When abdominal symptoms such as widespread persistent discomfort, ' wind ', nausea and anorexia were prominent, popular organic labels were the ptoses, hyperchlorhydria, chronic constipation, and intestinal auto-intoxication. Whatever the symptoms, they were often ultimately attributed to the malign influence of focal sepsis, and such diagnoses as a focal infection of a tooth, chronic tonsillitis and chronic cervicitis would follow. Even impotence, frigidity, dyspareunia and other sexual symptoms were attributed to inflammation of the seminal vesicles, lack of secretion from Bartholin's glands, or a congenitally small vagina. Indeed, perhaps the only somatic symptom of emotional origin which was not wrongly attributed to organic disease was weeping. Women so affected were not referred to the opthalmologist to be given the diagnosis of chronic inflammation of the lachrymal glands.

Even those doctors who recognized the possibility that somatic symptoms could have psychological causes were nevertheless apt to believe that a psychological diagnosis should only be made as a last resort, when all possibility of organic disease had been excluded. Patients were therefore subjected to long series of investigations in this exclusion process. This doctrine of diagnosis by exclusion is nonsensical, for it implies that if organic disease is found, the symptoms cannot be due to psychological causes. This explains some of the absurd diagnoses which were given to patients with psychosomatic symptoms. In the exclusion process it would be discovered that the patient had gastroptosis or a carious tooth, so the symptoms were attributed to these ' diseases ' (when there was a carious tooth by the mechanism of toxic absorption). In any case, it was and still is often impossible to exclude organic disease. This is notably true of coronary artery disease, cerebral glioma, and carcinoma of the body of the pancreas. The mechanistic physician after exhaustive tests going on for weeks might finally reach the absurd conclusion that a patient with one of these conditions must be neurotic.

A further reason for condemning this doctrine of diagnosing neurosis by exclusion is that many somatic symptoms are due to neither to psychological causes nor to any demonstrable organic lesion. This is true of migraine or premature systoles (which are considered below under the functional disorders).

Although this absurd doctrine has been widely condemned, it is still far from dead. Perhaps especially when patients have digestive symptoms many doctors are unwilling to conclude that these are psychosomatic, fearing that there may be some occult malignant disease. Such disease may, indeed, always be present, even in people who have no symptoms at all, but this cannot explain numerous and indefinite symptoms which have been present for years - the kind of symptoms which are in truth psychosomatic.

An important reason for concluding that symptoms are psycho-somatic is the existence of a clear relationship between the symptoms and the emotional state. To demonstrate this relationship, the patient should be looked at as a whole person and the doctor should inquire into his personal relationships and his problems, hopes and fears. In this way it may be evident that the somatic symptoms become worse when anxieties are worse. The subject with cardiac symptoms may, in worrying situations, develop palpitation, aching in the chest, unsteadiness and difficulty in breathing, whereas when he exercises he does not become distressed. Yet to this day many doctors fail to look at the patient as a whole and concentrate their attention on the presenting somatic symptoms and the organ or region whence the symptoms arise. This is especially true of some specialists. The ENT surgeon who is referred a patient with headache to 'exclude an ENT cause' may take the patient into a dark room to transilluminate his sinuses and send him to the X-ray department. But he may fail entirely to talk to the patient about his headache, his other symptoms, and his circumstances. And if he does discover some abnormality in his region he may wrongly attribute the headache to this.

Certain symptoms are characteristically, though not invariably, psychosomatic. Among them are weeping, trembling, impotence, dyspareunia, palpitation, sighing respiration or difficulty in ' filling the lungs ', a feeling of pressure in the head or a ' tight band ', general weakness and exhaustion. And as a rule a brief discussion with the patient leaves no doubt that these symptoms are in fact of emotional origin. Patients with psychosomatic symptoms typically have multiple complaints. When, in addition, these symptoms have been present for many months or years and especially if they are said to be continuous there are further grounds for concluding that they are psychosomatic.

One more reason for condemning the doctrine of diagnosis by exclusion is that patients with organic disease are especially liable to suffer psychosomatic symptoms. When a man is informed that he has heart disease, this is bound to upset him psychologically. And when he is also advised to make all sorts of restrictions to his life and a few decades ago this kind of advice was generally given, the degree of upset will probably be great. He may become aware of left mammary aching, rapid heart beat and palpitation, difficulty in breathing, and giddy sensations. He will easily take it for granted that these symptoms are due to his diseased heart, and may go into a vicious circle. The more symptoms he gets the worse will his worries be; the worse his emotional state becomes, the worse will be his symptoms. In this situation categorical reassurance by the doctor that the symptoms are due, not to the diseased heart, but to anxiety may undoubtedly give relief.

PSYCHOSOMATIC DISEASES

It has long been taken for granted by ordinary people that emotional upsets, as well as causing somatic symptoms, may also cause actual disease. In the novels read by our grandparents a miscarriage did not just happen by accident; it was brought on by some violent emotional storm. Those who were crossed in love might go into a fatal 'decline', the sudden arrival of bad news might bring on a stroke, a shock might be followed by 'brain fever' (whatever that was) and grief might cause a fatal 'broken heart'.

Reading history books, too, we are repeatedly told that all

manner of famous people were made ill or were sent to their deaths by emotional crises. A.L. Rowse[1] writes: 'The Younger Pitt returned to power in 1804 . . . to carry its burden virtually alone . . . (he) knew that it would cost him his life . . . he was forty-six, utterly worn out'. 'George VI had died in 1952 . . . worn out by work, the strain of war-years, of service to the country'. 'The strain of that year was too much (for Winston Churchill); in July he had a severe stroke'. According to A.J.P. Taylor (*New Statesman*, 26 October 1973) 'the strains of the Second World War were too much for many men. The War killed (President) Roosevelt'. And Aeneas Mackay[2] writes of James V of Scotland: 'When the news (of Solway Moss) reached James at Lochmaben, the melancholy which had been growing overwhelmed him and though he went to bed he could not rest . . . on 8 December Mary of Guise gave birth to Mary Stuart at Linlithgow. This news he treated as the last blow of an adverse fate, and exclaimed, "the Devil go with it. It will end as it began. It came with a lass, and will go with a lass". He spoke few sensible words after, and died on 16 December'.

Whenever politicians become ill or die, at least from non-infective conditions, the newspapers usually take it for granted that their illnesses were brought on by the strains of their unnatural lives. Stafford Cripps, Ernest Bevin, and Anthony Crosland were all said to have been killed by overwork. And in 1978 John Davies' sudden illness was attributed to the pressures even of being in opposition, and Sir Arthur Irvine's heart attack was said to have been brought on by his difficulties with his constituency party.

Nevertheless, during my student days in the thirties there was little mention of emotional factors in the aetiology of organic diseases. There was often reference to 'strain', it is true, but this appeared to be a physical rather than a psychological state. But during and after the war the concept of 'psychosomatic' diseases became increasingly popular. In the van of this movement was Flanders Dunbar, who published her celebrated *Emotions and Bodily Changes* in 1938.

Among the diseases which were said to be 'psychosomatic' were all those related to arteriosclerosis, and coronary thrombosis in particular, rheumatoid arthritis, 'fibrositis' and other rheumatic conditions, peptic ulcer, colitis and Crohn's disease, asthma, and migraine. Many of these maladies had previously been attributed to toxic absorption from septic foci. Emotional factors were also said to play a part in, if not to cause, some infections, including tuberculosis, and even many kinds of malignant disease. These ideas spread to the health conscious laity, and there were repeated references in newspapers and magazines to the high pressure executive with his ulcer or his coronary.

The bald assertion that some disease is 'psychosomatic' implies that it is at least largely, if not wholly, caused by emotional factors. But hard evidence that any of the conditions mentioned should be given this name has not been advanced. There are no good grounds for attributing rheumatoid arthritis to the emotions. Many patients who were considered to have 'fibrositis' complained of pain which was psychosomatic, but here the error lay in hypothesizing the organic disease 'fibrositis'. Coronary artery disease is closely involved with the emotions, as a heart attack is a horrifying experience, while emotional upsets can undoubtedly bring on anginal pain. But all this supplies no proof that the emotions can actually be responsible for disease of the coronary arteries. Emotional factors appear to play some part in the exacerbations of duodenal ulcer and possibly of colitis, but in many patients there is no evidence that these factors are important. Some attacks of asthma and of migraine are without doubt precipitated by the emotions, but other attacks in the same patients and all attacks in other patients do not appear to be psychosomatic.

With the possible exception of 'dermatitis artefacta' no organic disease can properly be given the unqualified label 'psychosomatic'. On the other hand, emotional factors may play an important part in the aetiology of many organic conditions, as well as those mentioned above. In a sense the venereal diseases are psychosomatic. The same is true of cirrhosis of the liver and other disorders of alcoholism and even of the carcinoma of bronchus which follows upon heavy smoking. Both obesity and the cachexia of 'anorexia nervosa' are largely psychosomatic. And many, perhaps most, road accidents and some other accidents are due more to emotional factors than to anything else, whether or not they are related to alcohol.

Although the psyche plays such a large part in causing somatic symptoms and although emotional factors are important in the aetiology of some organic conditions, the psychosomatic theory of disease has, then, been greatly oversold by enthusiasts. And in recent years we have heard less of so-called 'psychosomatic diseases' than we did 20 years ago. The desire to explain illness has always been so great that enthusiasm for some theory of aetiology has repeatedly lead to unjustified conclusions. In the 19th century masturbation provided a universal explanation of insanity. The toxic absorption theory, on the altar of which innumerable patients suffered extraction of teeth and removal of tonsils and other organs, was based entirely on flimsy theorizing and anecdotal cures. 30 or so years ago the General Adaption Syndrome of Hans Selye, which explained many maladies, had a brief vogue. In truth, solid knowledge about aetiology is meagre indeed.

FUNCTIONAL DISORDERS

The usual definition of a functional disorder is a disorder of function in an organ which is not diseased. This invites the question: 'How can we ever be certain that an organ is free of disease'? The answer is that we cannot. Nevertheless, recurrent disturbances may persist for years or for life in people who, when free of these disturbances, appear to be consistently well and there is absolutely no reason to suppose that the organ affected by the disturbances is diseased. Familiar examples of such disorders are migraine, epilepsy, dysmenorrhoea, proctalgia fugax and premature systoles.

The immediate cause of migraine is believed to be a temporary disturbance of some cerebral vessels. However frequent are the attacks, and however long they persist, there never develops demonstrable disease of the cerebral arteries. The immediate basis of epilepsy is said to be a disturbance in the chemico-electrical activity of the brain, though statements of this kind are of no help in understanding the nature of epilepsy. Much epilepsy is idiopathic and however long the attacks continue, the brain appears normal. Other epilepsy is symptomatic and clearly related to some disease affecting the brain. Dysmenorrhoea can be associated with uterine disease but in the vast majority of cases the uterus appears normal. Proctalgia fugax is a recurrent rectal pain attributed to spasm of the levator ani and occurring occasionally for years in susceptible subjects. Premature systoles are said to be commoner in association with some kinds of heart disease than in normal subjects, but they are frequent in young people in whom there is no suspicion of disease.

When attacks of epilepsy begin for the first time in association with a cerebral tumour, the epilepsy is not functional according to the usual definition. Yet it is still a temporary disturbance of function and is not related to the cerebral tumour in the same way as are such manifestations as dysphasia, hemiparesis, or hemianopia. The same considerations apply to the other conditions mentioned, which may have some connection with organic disease; they are still temporary disturbances of function. This category of functional disorders is, therefore, most useful. But it should be defined just as a disorder of function, without reference to the presence or absence of organic disease.

Although the maladies I have been discussing are in practice sometimes described as functional disorders, the somatic manifestations of emotional disorder are also said to be functional. We often hear of 'functional overlay' or occasionally just of 'overlay'. When a neurologist decrees that a patient's symptoms are 'purely functional', he usually means that they are hysterical. A patient with 'functional overlay' implies someone who has some apparently trivial organic disease but is making a great deal of fuss about it. Functional deafness means hysterical deafness. Emotional tachycardia may be described as functional tachycardia.

This use of the same word to describe quite different manifestations is unfortunate and leads to confusion. The most satisfactory way of resolving the problem is to confine the word functional to such conditions as migraine and premature systoles. Hysterical deafness, weakness, anaesthesia, or aphonia should be described as such. Emotional tachycardia, diarrhoea, sweating, or frequency of micturition should be called emotional. And the patient with a trivial disease who complains of a long list of symptoms, most of which can bear no relation to the disease, should be said to have psychological disorder as well as the trivial disease, not 'functional overlay'.

SUMMARY

(1) Many somatic symptoms are due to psychological causes. In the recent past, and to some extent now, such symptoms have been wrongly attributed to organic disease.

(2) Symptoms should be deemed psychosomatic, not because organic disease has been excluded, but for positive reasons. Patients with certain organic diseases are especially liable to have associated psychosomatic symptoms.

(3) Emotional factors may play some part in the aetiology of certain organic disease. But virtually no disease should be described baldly as psychosomatic.

(4) The functional disorders are such conditions as migraine, when there is a temporary disorder of function, usually unrelated to organic disease. Psychogenic symptoms are also commonly described as functional; this practice is deprecated.

References

1. Rowse, A.L. (1958). *The Later Churchills*. (London: Macmillan)
2. Mackay, Aeneas. *Dictionary of National Biography* (London: Oxford University Press)

4

Prevention

That prevention is better than cure is a truism. Doctors have often been accused of taking little interest in prevention, concentrating instead on 'established disease'. Is this condemnation justified? And can we do more than we have done to prevent disease?

In the affluent countries many diseases which used to be widespread, and are still widespread in the Third World, have virtually disappeared. We rarely see deficiency states (except among those with psychological disorder, such as anorexia nervosa or alcoholism). Many severe bacterial infections, including puerperal fever, enteric fever, cholera and diphtheria and many viral infections, notably smallpox and poliomyelitis, are extinct or nearly so and tuberculosis and syphilis are uncommon.

The maladies which are most obviously preventible in the affluent world are those related to indulgence. Many people overeat and most take little exercise. More than one third smoke and many get through 30 or 40 cigarettes daily. The consumption of alcohol has been rising and many people are badly addicted. A high proportion of injuries and deaths in road accidents are related to alcohol and many that are not so related are due to dangerous driving.

Individual doctors dealing with individual patients can no doubt do something to lessen these indulgence-related maladies. People who are urged by a doctor to stop smoking are more likely to do so than when urged by a lay person. Indeed, when a heavy smoker has been acutely ill, especially from a coronary thrombosis, there is an excellent chance that he will stop smoking completely for a time and a fair chance that he will never smoke again. But although this may give worthwhile gain, the only sensible course is never to start to smoke. The individual doctor can do nothing to achieve that goal.

Many doctors spend a lot of time in urging people to eat less sweets, starches, and fats. But they give this advice to patients who are already fat. And their success rate in persuading people to make a life-long reduction in their food intake is very small. Indeed, although obesity is eminently curable in the sense that if patients will only adopt the recommended treatment their weight will fall to normal and remain normal, we all know that in practice there are few more hopeless problems than the woman who has been grossly overweight for years. No condition better exemplifies the dictum 'prevention is better than cure' than does obesity. People achieve this goal of prevention by eating less as they grow older and never develop middle-aged spread. But all this has nothing to do with the individual doctor dealing with the individual patient. People who have always been thin do not seek interviews with their GPs and ask how they can continue to remain thin.

The medical profession as a whole is attacked, both by doctors and by the laity, for not taking any interest in alcohol addiction. We have often been informed that the average GP believes that he has one or two alcoholics on his list, whereas in fact he has perhaps 10 or 15. And we are urged to treat alcoholics 'early', while they are still doing a proper job, instead of waiting until they have degenerated to vagrancy and hopelessness. We are also repeatedly told to consider alcoholism as a 'disease', not as a state of moral degeneracy. But I have yet to see evidence that seeking out 'early' alcoholics and giving the most energetic treatment is, in the long run, of proven value. Suppose that a GP, anxious to do his bit in the fight against alcohol, hires a number of assistants who frequent the local pubs and observe his patients. In this way he discovers that, say, ten people on his list are drinking to excess. What can he do with this knowledge? Should he write to each patient and give him a surgery appointment? Or should he call on the spouses and discuss the situation with them? Most patients would probably consider all this as unwarrantable interference and if given an appointment would not keep it.

In general, the only alcohol addict that the doctor can help is the one who accepts that he is an addict and asks to be helped. And even then we all know that the success rate is small. Very few alcoholics ever become moderate drinkers and not many become permanently teetotal - the only state recommended by Alcoholics Anonymous. Most people with a drinking problem pretend to their relatives, colleagues, and doctors, and even try to convince themselves, that they have no such problem. Only when they have advanced far along the road is there much chance that they will accept that their addiction to alcohol is beyond control.

In so far as action can be taken to combat smoking, excessive drinking, overeating, and under-exercising, this should be taken much more on behalf of society as a whole than by the individual efforts of doctors dealing with their individual patients. Such action can have a considerable impact.

LEGISLATION AND PROPAGANDA

The simplest and most effective means of reducing tobacco and alcohol consumption is to raise the price. Each time the Chancellor of the Exchequer increases the tobacco duty the sale of cigarettes drops, if only temporarily, and a few people cease to smoke permanently. No doubt a really large increase in duty would be followed by a correspondingly large increase in the number of non-smokers. It has been suggested that the Government should announce that there will be a specified increase at each budget for the foreseeable future.

As Kendell[1] (1979) has pointed out, by comparison with the average income, the cost of alcohol has greatly declined in Britain. 'Between 1950 and 1976 the length of time a male manual worker had to work to pay for a pint of beer fell from 23 minutes to 12; the work time to pay for a bottle of whisky fell from 6½ hours to 2. The time needed to pay for a large loaf increased during this period from 9 minutes to 11'. Kendell also comments: 'The available evidence strongly suggests that (alcoholism and total alcohol consumption) are closely linked'. If the price of alcoholic drinks were doubled, there would be a sharp drop in alcohol consumption. Although it has been said that this would have little effect on the bad addict (who would still go on drinking as much but neglect his family more and get even worse into debt), there can be no doubt that there would be nonetheless a corresponding decrease in the number of alcohol addicts.

An important secondary effect of massive increases in the price of tobacco and alcohol would be the increase in the money available for spending by Government agencies. Although in Britain taxation has not been linked to specific expenditure, it could well be argued that since the reason for the increased duties is to improve health, some at least of the money could properly be spent on the National Health Service. As to whether or not the way to improve the National Health Service is to spend more on it is a matter which will be discussed in Chapter 5.

Since it has been generally accepted that smoking is largely responsible for lung cancer and chronic bronchitis and plays a part in the aetiology of many other maladies, there has been a moderate amount of propaganda to dissuade people, and especially the young, from smoking. There has also been a ban on cigarette advertising on TV and on the packets of all tobacco products there is a health warning. More widespread propaganda and a total ban on all kinds of tobacco advertising would, without reasonable doubt, lessen tobacco consumption further. But as to whether or not this is justified is hotly debated, though I believe that it is justified. It can be argued that Government is entitled to put before the public the facts about the damage done by tobacco, but beyond that the public should make up its own mind.

Some of the damage done by smoking is to unfortunate non-smokers who are forced to inhale smoke in public places. Legislation to ban smoking is held, by its opponents, to be unreasonable interference with the rights of the individual, but to me it seems entirely reasonable that there should be a total ban on smoking in shops, banks, etc. and that wherever practicable there should be smoke-free zones in restaurants and cinemas and smoke-free bars in pubs. We can perhaps hope that in time it will become generally accepted that only when consenting adults are meeting in private should smoking be tolerated.

Although by far the most important cause of lung cancer and

chronic bronchitis is smoking, other kinds of atmospheric pollution also contribute, especially to bronchitis. Workers in certain dusty occupations, notably miners in some areas, are liable to chest diseases largely due to noxious inhaled substances. Legislation has already reduced atmospheric pollution very greatly and has improved the situation in dusty work places. We can anticipate that further legislation, designed to lessen in particular sulphur dioxide and unburnt hydrocarbons, will improve the situation even more.

Propaganda appears to be ineffective in persuading people to drink moderately; the majority do so without benefit of propaganda and the minority of alcohol addicts are insusceptible. But propaganda has been widely directed to those who drink and drive. Since the most common cause of death in young adults is accident, especially road accident, and since many of those involved in accidents have been drinking heavily, this is a most important matter. When the breathalyser was first introduced there was a dramatic fall in the number of road accidents, especially in the evenings after closing time. But as the years have gone by more and more people have been driving with excessive levels of blood alcohol. Propaganda, however persistent and widespread, is unlikely to have much effect. The only effective means of improving the situation is stronger legislation. In Sweden, we understand, legislation has been so fierce that few people take the risk of driving after drinking. Similar legislation in Britain would be violently opposed as a gross interference with liberty, but if, as there is very reason to suppose, it would greatly reduce death and maiming on the road, it would, I believe, be justified.

There has been much other legislation designed to reduce road accidents, such as the laying down of minimum thickness of tread on tyres and the annual test on older cars. One measure of proven value in lessening the severity of injuries from road accidents is the wearing of seat-belts. All cars are compulsorily fitted with belts and there has been endless propaganda urging people to use them. However, most people in Britain still do not do so. In most other countries the wearing of seat-belts by drivers and front seat passengers is compulsory. In spite of all the opposition to this measure in Britain, we may anticipate that a law compelling people to use seat-belts will be passed before long - a law which seems wholly justified.

Before the 20th century the great majority of people even in the most affluent societies took much exercise. The work of many involved continuous physical toil and most of those doing sedentary jobs walked considerable distances every day to and from work. But as machinery has replaced man-power at work and motor cars have obviated the need to walk, many people have virtually ceased to exercise. The typical modern man walks a few yards to his car after breakfast, drives to an office or factory, sits there all day, drives back home and spends the evenings slumped in a chair half looking at the Box. At the weekend, for a change, he drives the family to the country and sits by the car having a picnic.

There is good evidence that this modern lack of exercise plays a part in causing coronary artery disease and other maladies and it also encourages obesity, which in turn increases various health risks. There has been little official propaganda urging people to take exercise and no legislation to compel them to do so. Legislation is out of the question, but would propaganda be justified? It seems to be proper that the authorities should inform people that exercise is beneficial but beyond that the public should draw its own conclusions. On the other hand, the authorities could rightly provide more facilities for people to exercise, especially in the large cities.

Since it became widely accepted by the health-conscious public that exercise is beneficial there has been an increase in exercise-taking by the sedentary population. Jogging in particular has become popular, and in the United States (where fashions are set which are later followed by the rest of the affluent world) there has been a jogging craze, though we understand that this is now on the decline. And some evidence has been advanced that exercise of a degree to cause marked dyspnoea, such as jogging, is more beneficial than even prolonged exercise, such as walking, which does not.

This recent reversal of the trend in the affluent world to less and less exercise can only be applauded. But one may wonder whether many people will continue to force themselves to exercise indefinitely as a means to health unless they enjoy taking the exercise. And many people do enjoy it by playing golf, tennis, and other games or by country walks. The provision by the authorities of facilities for games increases the number of people who exercise.

When exercise becomes a habit, continuing to take it indefinitely never becomes a burden. The simplest way of exercising as a habit is to walk the whole or part of the way to and from work. People who achieve this habit may continue in the same way until they retire and they derive an immediate sense of well-being as well as a diminished liability to various maladies.

Food has long been the subject of legislation. Most of this has been to safeguard the public from infection and deficiency states and some of it to safeguard the animals who provide the food. Many people eat too much and there is also a widely held opinion among the experts that many eat wrongly. Two especially common food faults are said to be that food contains too little roughage and in particular too little bran and too much sugar and animal fats. Should legislation or propaganda attempt to correct these faults?

Legislation has already compelled people to eat additives in certain foods, such as iron and vitamins in bread, although there is no clear evidence that most people would come to harm if they were omitted. This compulsory medication has caused no protests. No doubt if it was illegal to sell other than 100% wholemeal bread the health of the population would improve by a lessening of the incidence of diverticular disease and perhaps appendicitis and varicose veins. Nevertheless, since so many people prefer white bread the attempt to compel them not to eat it is unjustified. Moreover, any such attempt would provoke violent opposition. Propaganda which points out the benefits of wholemeal bread, on the other hand, seems quite proper.

One of the most hotly debated aspects of food in recent years has been the animal fat content. Those people who eat much animal fat have been shown to have higher cholesterol and other lipid levels in their blood than do those who eat little of such fat. And people with these higher levels are unduly liable to coronary thrombosis. In consequence, doctors (especially in the United States) have widely advised patients to reduce the animal fat content of their food. There has nevertheless been no clear evidence that the liability to coronary thrombosis is reduced by this measure. There is therefore no justification at present for official propaganda to persuade people to eat less animal fat (See also Chapter 8, p. 153).

Two common dietary faults are to eat too many calories and too much sugar. The excess sugar usually accounts for much of the excessive calorie intake but is also believed to be largely responsible for caries in teeth. There can be no question of legislation to compel people to correct these errors. There seems no objection on principle to propaganda which urges them to do so, but it seems highly unlikely that any amount of propaganda would persuade people to eat less calories. Propaganda which merely stressed the risks of excessive sugar intake might well, on the other hand, have some success.

The fluoride story illustrates some of the difficulties faced by legislators when they attempt to compel people to change what they swallow. There is overwhelming evidence that if drinking water contains one part per million of fluoride the incidence of dental caries is greatly reduced. And there is absolutely no evidence that fluoride in this quantity does harm. In consequence, doctors' and dentists' organizations have repeatedly urged the fluoridation of water supplies and successive Secretaries of State for Social Services have given their support. But the anti-fluoride lobby has so far succeeded in preventing most water undertakings from adding fluoride. Why this particular measure should arouse such passionate feeling is not apparent to me. No-one objects to the compulsory addition of chlorine to prevent water-borne infections, and this can affect the quality of the water, whereas no-one can tell that fluoride has been added. The anti-fluoride enthusiasts claim that there is some profound difference between adding chlorine and adding fluoride to water. Thus, in a letter to the *Guardian* (12 January, 1979) Professor H.M. Sinclair said: 'The difference in principle should be obvious: chlorine is added to make water safe to drink; fluoride is added as a form of mass medication . . . this is an entirely new principle since everyone has a right to a non-medicated water supply'. But if it is said that 'chlorine is added to prevent water-borne infections and fluoride is added to prevent dental caries', this profound difference in principle is made to disappear. Those who are opposed to fluoridation also repeatedly claim that fluoride is a 'poison'. If fluoride is taken in large amounts it is indeed poisonous, just as is sodium choride and any other salt. Yet no-one has suggested that the fluoride should be removed from those water supplies in which it occurs naturally. There is apparently a world of difference between one part per million of fluoride provided by nature and the same amount provided by man.

The anti-fluoride lobby are a small minority. If they can only be overborn the dental state of the nation would without doubt improve. And those who feel so passionately should be able to obtain the means to remove the fluoride from their own water.

VACCINATION

Much of the diminution in the incidence of certain infections can be attributed to vaccination. This is especially true of diphtheria and poliomyelitis. On the other hand, the diminution in tuberculosis appears to be due much more to the isolation and effective treatment of the infective subjects of the disease than to vaccination, though the incidence of tuberculosis had been falling for a long time before we had effective treatment.

Vaccination would be the perfect means of prevention if it were both totally effective and wholly devoid of risk. For many infections it is highly effective, but unfortunately it always carries some risk. And there have been occasional large-scale disasters from improperly made vaccine. Recently there have been numerous references to brain damage allegedly caused by whooping cough vaccine, though there is much doubt as to whether many or most of the affected children were in fact damaged by the vaccine. This scare has unfortunately been accompanied by a drop in all kinds of vaccination, as well as in whooping cough vaccination.

The individual doctor dealing with his own patients is very much concerned with vaccination, as he is the obvious person to whom anxious parents turn to ask the question 'should my child be vaccinated against a specified infection, and especially against whooping cough?' This can put him in a difficult position, since he can hardly deny that there is a faint risk of brain damage. There is no easy solution to this problem, but the doctor's best course probably is to emphasize that the risk is exceedingly small. Should he give a definite advice for or against vaccination, or should he put the facts as he knows them before the parents and tell them they must make up their own minds? Different doctors give different answers to this question and, no doubt, sometimes a doctor's answer will be influenced by the personalities of the parents concerned.

The main means of encouraging vaccination is, nevertheless, not through the individual doctor but by legislation and propaganda. Over the years there has been a great deal of propaganda urging people (or their children) to be vaccinated. And actual vaccination has often been carried out at infant welfare and school clinics. Years ago legislation made smallpox vaccination compulsory, though parents who were opposed could always sign a form to say that they had a conscientious objection to it. Now, as smallpox is extinct apart from one small area of Africa, there can be no good ground to recommend it, since the risk of the vaccination must be much greater than the risk of developing the disease. It is now difficult to conceive of circumstances which could justify legislation to make any kind of vaccination compulsory (except, perhaps, for certain immigrants). The one proper means of encouraging it is propaganda.

THE REGULAR MEDICAL EXAMINATION

The one means of prevention which necessarily involves the individual doctor dealing with individual people is the regular medical examination. In the United States many doctors spend much of their time in this activity. In Britain some GPs do certain particular observations, such as blood-pressure estimation, on patients who are attending for other reasons. A few enthusiastic GPs have even encouraged all of certain categories of patient, such as men between the ages of 30 and 60, to attend specifically for blood pressure and perhaps other estimations. But if a patient makes an appointment with a GP and tells him 'I feel perfectly well but I would like a medical examination' few GPs would agree to do this.

A regular medical examination can consist of anything from one single observation (such as blood-pressure estimation or cervical smear) to the most elaborate battery of tests. Both in America and Europe the trend has been to more and more elaboration, especially since the development of machines which simultaneously carry out numerous blood estimations. In addition to these and a complete physical examination, the full procedure is likely to include at least a chest X-ray, a 12 lead electrocardiograph and microscopic and chemical studies of the urine. There may also be a barium-meal and barium enema studies and perhaps endoscopy. One can easily envisage that as the years go by more and more tests will be added. Perhaps before long complete body scans by computer-assisted tomography will become part of the routine for the high American executive. In Britain, this kind of activity is mainly confined to the senior employees of large corporations. The studies are paid for by the corporations and are mostly carried out by BUPA.

The ordinary man will naturally assume that, since important people are offered regular medical examinations, this must do them good. Indeed, it may appear obvious that if a regular service for a £10,000 company car is recommended every 3 months, it must surely be right that a high executive (who is worth many times more than a car) should also have his service. This analogy is actually used to justify and encourage regular examinations. In addition, those doctors who take part in the procedure are naturally in favour of it and if a doctor, who is the expert on human bodies, advises that regular elaborate tests are desirable, he should, the public will conclude, know what he is talking about.

The first part of the procedure usually consists of history-taking and physical examination. These may reveal that the subject has various worries about his family or work and he may admit to smoking, to unwise drinking, to overeating and to taking no exercise. Examination may perhaps show obesity, carious teeth or pyorrhoea, hallux valgus, varicose veins, ingrowing toe-nail and hypertension.

With the possible exception of hypertension, a regular examination is not needed to bring these points to light. The subject will already be aware that he smokes, drinks too much, eats too much, takes no exercise, is overweight, has varicose veins, and is worried. It has nevertheless been said that some people will accept advice at a regular medical to improve their habits, although they will not make an appointment to see their own GP to ask his advice. But there is no clear evidence that this is so. And it seems most improbable that a man who has been smoking heavily for years and is much overweight will suddenly stop smoking and permanently reduce his food-intake just because he has attended for a regular examination. And if he has varicose veins, hallux valgus, or a variety of other innocent conditions, to advise 'treatment' when the subject is not complaining is ridiculous. On the contrary, when a patient sees his own GP actually complaining of varicose veins, to which he may attribute aching in the legs, the right course is often to advise no action, pointing out that the veins are doing no harm and are not responsible for the leg ache. If he has carious teeth, it may seem reasonable to suggest that he sees a dentist, but there is no evidence that attending to his teeth will improve his state of health.

The one common abnormality brought to light by a routine physical examination is hypertension. In the past there was no benefit from this, as no useful action could be taken. But we can now reduce the blood pressure with drugs without usually causing unpleasant side effects. And without reasonable doubt reducing markedly elevated blood pressure improves the outlook, especially in young men.

Although the discovery of markedly elevated blood pressure in a young man is likely to benefit him, most hypertension is mild or moderate and is found in the middle-aged or elderly. Treatment for such people is of unknown value. And if someone is told that his blood pressure is high, various ill effects are likely to follow. Even if the doctor is reassuring, the subject can hardly fail to be at least somewhat alarmed. For every one knows that people with raised blood pressure are liable to strokes and other disasters. As a consequence of his anxiety the subject may develop unpleasant sensations in the head such as flushings, dizziness and pressure, perhaps also with palpitation and aching in the chest. Those who become aware that they have hypertension are liable to miss work more often than they did. Stewart[2] (1953) compared two groups of people with similar degrees of hypertension, some of whom knew and the others did not know their blood pressures were raised. Only three of the 104 unaware patients complained of headache (though others admitted to it when asked leading questions) whereas 71 of the 96 who knew they had hypertension did so.

Even the discovery of hypertension may, therefore, often do more harm than good. And if the doctor does discover hypertension, but decides that no action is indicated because of the age of the patient or the moderate rise of pressure, he may reasonably withhold information to the patient about his blood pressure. This is a matter which often arouses strong feelings among the health-conscious public, who insist that they have no wish to be

treated as helpless children by the medical profession and have a
'right to know' if anything is amiss. When someone goes to a doctor
with symptoms, and the doctor discovers why he has these
symptoms, as a rule he should explain what he has found, though
even here there may be exceptions, such as the discovery of
hopeless malignant disease. But when a doctor discovers some
abnormality which is not responsible for symptoms and does not
require treatment he is usually doing his best for the patient by
withholding his discovery.

URINE TESTING

The abnormality in the urine most often discovered at a regular
medical examination is sugar, and this usually implies diabetes.
There are, indeed, many unsuspected diabetics. Nearly all are
middle-aged or elderly and most are obese. Enthusiasts have
carried out diabetes detection drives. But there is little evidence
that discovering diabetes improves the patient's prospects by
lessening the incidence of retinopathy, nephropathy, gangrene, and
other complications. If the patient is overweight (as he usually is) he
should reasonably be urged to make a permanent reduction in his
calorie intake. And the same advice should be given to the
overweight non-diabetic. This advice is rarely followed. On the
other hand, if someone is told that he has diabetes he may stop
eating sweets and having sugar in tea or coffee, as everyone 'knows'
that sugar is poisonous to diabetics. He may also change from white
to brown bread. But the likelihood of his sharply reducing his total
calorie intake for the rest of his life is small. Some of those
discovered to have diabetes have been prescribed sulphonyl urea
compounds. This is nearly always a mistake. Even though a
restricted diet is also advised, the patient is apt to assume that
because he is having tablets this makes dieting less important. In
consequence, he puts on more weight.

ELECTROCARDIOGRAPHY

The electrocardiograph seems to have an especial appeal to the health-conscious public and the 12 lead e.c.g. tracing is an important part of the executive's regular examination.

Patients with various kinds of advanced heart disease, and in particular with coronary artery disease causing angina of effort, may have normal resting e.c.g.s. After exercise, e.c.g.s may then show abnormalities, but even a normal post-exercise e.c.g. does not prove that the coronary circulation is satisfactory. The e.c.g. is also worthless as an index of prognosis; many executives who have emerged from their regular medical with everything normal have later dropped dead from coronary artery disease.

E.c.g. abnormalities are sometimes found in symptom-free people. The commonest of these are premature systoles; others are inverted T waves, left and right axis deviation and left and right bundle-branch block. What action should be taken if these are found? If the subject is told that he has some abnormality, he can hardly fail to be worried, even if he is reassured that the abnormality is not serious. It is in any case usually impossible to know just what significance these abnormalities have and experts notoriously disagree. A *British Medical Journal* leading article[4] (1970) comments:'There is a low incidence of right or left BBB among an otherwise healthy, non-patient population ... it is this situation which faces the practitioner with a dilemma ... It is justifiable to strongly reassure such a subject rather than to court the risk of undue cardiac invalidism'. But if the subject is never told that he has an abnormality, there can be no risk of 'undue cardiac invalidism'. And I am aware of no e.c.g. abnormality discovered in a symptom-free patient which justifies any action.

The electrocardiograph, therefore, so far from giving useful information at a regular medical examination, is the most fatuous of all the tests done on these occasions. For a normal e.c.g. can co-exist with advanced heart disease and nothing useful can be done if an abnormality is found. I should never agree to having an e.c.g. done on myself when I felt well. 'Where ignorance is bliss tis folly to be wise'.

DISCOVERING CANCER 'EARLY'

An important reason for doing regular examinations is often said to be to discover cancer at an 'early, curable stage'. This is thought especially relevant to carcinoma of the cervix uteri, because of the occurrence of cancer *in situ,* and to less extent of carcinoma of the breast. All over the Western World vast numbers of women have had regular cervical smears and it has been suggested that there should be special mammography clinics at which women are advised to attend at intervals.

Many surgeons also repeatedly emphasize the importance of discovering cancer 'early'. We hear depressing accounts of women who have delayed and delayed to take advice while lumps in their breasts get bigger and bigger, or of men who have had dyspeptic symptoms for many months before being found to have inoperable carcinoma of the stomach, either because they failed to see their GPs or because their GPs treated them with alkali instead of referring them to hospital.

Although, other things being equal, the earlier most cancer is discovered the better, a far more important determinant of the prognosis of cancer than the age of the lesion is its inherent malignancy. By far the commonest cancer among men in Britain is carcinoma bronchus, and as a rule this is highly malignant. Frequently metastases develop before the primary growth is big enough either to cause symptoms or a shadow on the X-ray plate. If every smoker had a chest X-ray every 3 months as part of a drive to discover cancer 'early' this could not possibly have more than a marginal effect on the cancer death rate. Much the same is true of carcinoma of stomach. However quickly a patient seeks advice after developing the symptoms, or even if a growth is discovered on routine barium-meal, the prognosis is usually bad. The commonest neoplasm of the central nervous system is glioma, and nothing is gained by discovering it 'early'. On the other hand, many cancers of the large bowel and of the body of the uterus are comparatively benign', and even if they have been present for a long time the prognosis is often good. Chronic lymphatic leukaemia is quite often discovered by accident from blood counts done for other reasons than the suspicion of leukaemia. This 'early' discovery does not affect the outcome and treatment is rarely indicated.

The common cancer for which early discovery is usually held to be particularly important is carcinoma breast. Yet here too the natural malignancy clearly plays a large part in determining the outcome, and growths can metastasize while minute in size. There is, moreover, profound uncertainty as to the best means of treating this disease (whereas 40 years ago everyone 'knew' that the treatment for all kinds of early cancer of the breast was radical mastectomy).

The discovery of a pre-malignant condition is widely thought to be especially valuable, as the tissue can then be eradicated before malignancy develops. This is most relevant to the carcinoma *in situ*, which is so often found in the cervix uteri. If every case of invasive carcinoma cervix was preceded by carcinoma *in situ* which remained quiescent for several years, the finding of carcinoma *in situ* would indeed be profoundly important and regular examination would virtually guarantee that the individual would not die of carcinoma cervix. Unfortunately, the situation is not so simple. Although it has often been claimed that regular cervical cytology to detect carcinoma *in situ* will lower the death rate from carcinoma cervix, there is no unequivocal evidence that this is so. Many large-scale studies have been made, but the statistics have been conflicting. The overall incidence of carcinoma of the cervix has been falling for many years, both in the places where screening has been widely practised and those where it has not.

When attempts are being made to discover cancer 'early' and there are abnormal findings, these do not, unfortunately, always clearly indicate either malignancy or non-malignancy. A frequent finding in this quest is a shadow on the chest X-ray film. The radiologist habitually reports a shadow 'which must be considered malignant until proved otherwise', and this may either be in the lung field or hilar. This may put the clinician in a most difficult situation. If the shadow is hilar he will no doubt do a blood count and ESR, but if these are unhelpful and the patient is symptom-free he will probably decide that the best course is to re X-ray after an interval. What, then, should be said to the unfortunate patient? However often he is told that the situation looks in no way serious and there is no reason to suspect cancer, he will inevitably be worried. If after another 3 months the shadow is much the same, he will no doubt be reassured once more but told that to be on the safe side yet another X-ray should be taken in another 3 months. This uncertainty may continue for a long time. Yet whatever is causing the hilar shadow, the patient can hardly benefit from this 'early' discovery. If the shadow is due to sarcoidosis and he had never been X-rayed he would never have known there was anything wrong and have been spared all this anxiety. If the basis of the trouble is a reticulosis or other malignant condition treatment is not indicated in the absence of symptoms and there is also no gain from the early discovery.

If the shadow is in the lung field, sputum cytology and bronchoscopy may be done. If these are indeterminate, the decision may be made to await developments for a month or two and re-X-ray. Alternatively, a thoracotomy may be performed. If in fact the cause of the suspicious shadow is a carcinoma, the early discovery may have improved the prognosis, but if there are already metastases (as will often be so) there will be no gain. If the condition is in fact innocent, the shadow being due to an area of collapse or consolidation, nothing is gained and much is lost by starting along the road which begins with a chest X-ray taken routinely. Not only are the investigations and operations unpleasant. The subject and his relatives are given much anxiety, however much the doctor tries to reassure them. If the X-ray had never been taken the trouble would have cleared up spontaneously and all his distress would have been avoided.

The discovery of marked hypertension in young men is likely to do more good than harm. The same may be true of the discovery of carcinoma *in situ* from doing regular cervical smears, though this is unproven. There may sometimes be slight gain by discovering early cancer. And there are some other conditions, including pulmonary tuberculosis (though is most parts of Britain this is rarely found by routine X-rays), glaucoma, and, in infants, phenylketonuria and hypothyroidism, the discovery of which at a regular examination is worthwhile. But even in these situations there may be loss as well as gain. The least uncommon of these conditions, hypertension, is usually treated by life-long drugs and although there is fair chance that side-effects will not occur, the very fact of being put on life-long drugs may have a demoralizing effect on the sensitive person. There is also a risk that such a person will develop headache and other symptoms due to anxiety, even though the doctor does his best to reassure him.

The fact that a regular examination can be worthwhile in a few specified circumstances provides absolutely no justification for advocating such examinations in general. Any particular procedure for any particular category of person should be assessed separately on its own merits. To advocate multiphasic screening examinations on every one is nonsensical. In the modern world of medicine there is a vast amount of waste (which will be considered in Chapter 5 and 8). There is no worse example of waste than the performing of huge numbers of tests on as many of the population as can be persuaded to have them.

Those doctors who enthusiastically advocate regular medical examinations probably tend to advocate 'treatment' if any kind of abnormality is found, since this will tend to bolster their belief that the whole procedure is worth while. For if no action is taken on account of some abnormality this will imply that there was no point in discovering the abnormality. But, apart from the few conditions I have mentioned there is hardly ever justification for advising treatment if the patient is not complaining.

MEDICAL EXAMINATION IN RELATION TO WORK

Although people are increasingly encouraged to have regular examinations which are paid for by their employers, they are at least at liberty to refuse to avail themselves of this service. But in certain circumstances people are compelled to have a medical examination in connection with their work. This often happens before they are accepted by some corporation. A potential employee may be told that he has been accepted 'subject to medical examination' and later be informed that he has 'failed' the medical, so he cannot be accepted. From time to time one reads in the newspapers of these people. The following appeared in the *Guardian* of 23 August 1978, under the heading 'Healthy man who failed medical loses job'. 'He was examined by the company doctor and told he had hypertension (high blood pressure) . . . He has apparently no legal redress. He was not "unfairly dismissed" because the company only hired him subject to a medical and paid him off on the grounds that he failed to reach the required standard . . . the doctor who examined him said "I am sure (he) is fit for work, but we are not so· much concerned about his present health as his future health. The company has a generous sick benefit scheme and I am required only to allow A1 people on to the permanent staff'. During my medical career I saw many such unfortunates. Distressed and alarmed by their rejection they had naturally sought the advice of their GPs, who in turn referred them to me.

When a man is a candidate for a job which his ill-health may be a danger to others, his rejection is of course justified. Epileptics must not drive trains or pilot aeroplanes and typhoid carriers must not be cooks. Yet an ordinary medical examination, including electro-encephalograms, electrocardiograms and the most sophisticated X-rays, is of minimal help in detecting people who are likely to be a danger to others. If an epileptic chooses to lie about his attacks, no test can reveal the truth.

Drivers and pilots also have regular exhaustive tests every year or so throughout their careers and if something is found which in the opinion of the examining doctor makes them unduly liable to sudden incapacity, they may lose their jobs. No-one can object to this in principle, though in practice it is impossible to evaluate the hazard represented by some abnormality. Air pilots are liable to lose their licences on account of hypertension or of the development of an e.c.g. abnormality since the previous tracing. In so far as air disasters are due to human error, this error derives from the psyche immensely more often than from the sudden onset of bodily incapacity. However, if the examining doctor does have grounds for believing that a pilot has a condition making him even slightly liable to sudden incapacity, he cannot be blamed for recomending that the pilot is grounded.

In most situations the question of being a danger to others does not arise. The main reason why people are rejected medically is because the examining doctor believes that they may not give continuous service in the foreseeable future. The doctor who acts in this way is putting the supposed interests of his employer before the interests of his patient. I have suggested[4] (Todd, 1965) that the doctor then requires a modified version of the Hippocratic oath, such as: 'The regimen I adopt shall be for the benefit of my patients according to my ability and judgement and not for their hurt or for any wrong, unless I am examining them on behalf of an employer, when the welfare of the patient shall count for nothing, and the interests of the employer shall be my sole concern'.

If the doctor who does pre-employment medical examinations is justified in rejecting some candidate for a job, other doctors who work for other firms can reach the same conclusion. If pre-employment medical examinations became universal, unfortunate people with hypertension, diabetes, asthma, rheumatoid arthritis, peptic ulcer etc., might be unable to get any kind of job, and they and their families would have to be supported by the state. We often hear of those who are denied a fair chance of work because of their origins or colour. But we also hear of processions, petitions, and riots designed to put right this wrong. Those unfortunates who are rejected medically are a scattered and weak minority, and no-one riots to redress their wrongs.

In the complex modern world few problems have a simple solution. But the problem of medical rejection could easily be solved. Leaving aside those whose sudden incapacity may endanger others, I have long maintained[4] (Todd, 1965) that medical rejection should be made illegal. Failing this, doctors who do pre-employment medical examinations should refuse to put the interests of their employers before the interests of the individual. And if they are confronted with directives (such as that only people who are first-class insurance lives or those with blood pressures below a specified level should be taken on) they should either insist that these are altered or ignore them.

The doctor who casually rejects candidates for employment because they have a raised blood pressure, albuminuria, or a heart murmur would be well advised to consider how he would feel if he were treated in a similar manner. Suppose he is a senior registrar and that, after years of fruitless application for consultant appointments, he is finally made a consultant 'subject to medical examination'. After this, he is informed that because his blood-pressure is too high he cannot be made a consultant after all. Would his rage and despair be in any way lessened by the Chairman's kindly assurance: 'Although you are unfit to be a consultant, you will be allowed to stay on as a supernumerary registrar'?

SUMMARY

(1) In the affluent societies the chief preventible maladies are those related to indulgence, mainly smoking, overeating, excessive

drinking and under-exercising. The individual doctor can play little part in preventing them. Society as a whole, helped by legislation and propaganda, should take action. Pollution related maladies must also be dealt with by social action.

(2) Vaccination is valuable in preventing certain infections. Individual doctors can play a part by recommending this, but the main means of encouraging it is propaganda.

(3) The preventive measure which needs the individual doctor is regular medical examination. The benefits from this are very small; the potential ill effects are large.

(4) Doctors sometimes reject candidates for employment after a medical examination. Leaving aside those, such as air pilots, the sudden incapacity of whom may endanger others, this is never justified and should be made illegal.

References

1. Kendell, R.E. (1979). *Br. Med. J.*, **1**, 367
2. Stewart, I. Mc D.G. (1953). *Lancet*, **1**, 1261
3. Leading article (1970). *Br. Med. J.*, **1**, 450
4. Todd, J.W. (1965). *Lancet*, **1**, 797

5

The Right and Wrong Use of Resources

For many years we have heard the repeated complaint that more resources should be devoted to health in Britain. Nearly all the other advanced countries, we are told, spend more than we do. In the United States 8.6% of the GNP is devoted to health care, a figure that has been rising for years and on present trends will exceed 10% in the early 1980s, whereas in Britain we only spend about 6% of the GNP on health. We read article after article in both the lay and medical press about these matters. A leading article in *The Times,* 12 July, 1978 was entitled 'Sickness of the Health Service' and the situation was assessed in the light of the Chairman's address at the Annual Representative Meeting of the British Medical Association. In this address he claimed that 'standards were rapidly deteriorating, service was impersonal and inadequate, and the idealism of those who provided it was being dissipated by lack of resources'.

The supreme basis to all our difficulties is said to be enshrined in the phrase 'Infinite demand: finite resources'. Dr David Owen[1], then Minister of State (Health) at the DHSS, used this phrase in an article in the *Lancet* (1976), based on an address given to the East Kent Division of the BMA. Among his comments were: 'The two assumptions underlying the philosophy of the 1946 Act was that health need was finite and that, once need was identified, society would be willing to divert sufficient resources from other uses . . . to meet it. This philosophy has proved hopelessly wrong and demand, far from being finite, is now seen to approach the infinite'. The first of a series of six articles in *The Times* in 1978 by Annabel Ferriman[2], on the condition and outlook for the NHS appeared under the heading: 'Main Trouble is Infinite Demand for Treatment'. Among her statements were 'In recent years complaints that (the NHS) is "falling apart" from lack of money have become louder . . . But unless the public can cultivate a more realistic approach, live a healthier life and go to the doctor less, the service is likely to be pulled apart by competing claims for scarce resources'.

The public are, then, repeatedly blamed for demanding so much. In turn, the politicians are blamed for encouraging the public to make demands. *A British Medical Journal* leading article (1974) begins[3] 'The time has come for realism' and ends 'the politicians' claim that the NHS offered all available treatments to every patient was always something of a fraud, but now it is no longer possible even to go on pretending it'. And another *British Medical Journal* leading article[4] (1977) on the underfinancing of the NHS states: 'one aspect of the NHS that has long irritated doctors has been the regular emphasis on the "free" NHS by politicians, who have simultaneously extolled its comprehensive facilities'. As well as the politicians and the public, the bureaucracy is also blamed. The number of bureaucrats, we are endlessly told, was vastly increased in the NHS reorganization in 1974 and, bureaucrats being bureaucrats, they constantly interfere in the doctor-patient relationship and generally worsen the situation. Indeed, according to nearly all the doctors who write about these problems, just about the only people who deserve no blame for the dire straits into which the NHS has sunk are the doctors themselves.

The health services can be separated into the caring side and the curing side. The caring side deals with those unfortunate people who need an asylum because they cannot live independent lives. Here, the NHS overlaps with the social services, since when an old person becomes incapable of looking after himself there may be doubt as to whether he should be in a hospital or in a welfare home. There is also much overlap between caring and curing. An old person who needs care may also be helped by an operation. And many patients 'block acute beds' - how often we hear this phrase! - because they have been admitted as emergencies and never recover enough to be able to live independent lives.

As the average age of the population rises, more and more caring is needed. And at present there is a general shortage of caring accommodation. This intractable problem will be considered in Chapter 6.

GENERAL PRACTITIONER SERVICES

Although we hear *ad nauseam* about the demands of the public the only direct demand which patients can make on the NHS is to seek an interview with a GP or go to a casualty or VD department. Everything done beyond that is underwritten by some doctor.

On most occasions when someone sees a GP the only resource which should be consumed is the doctor's time. No prescription, no hospital referral and no investigation is needed. This is true of most people who attend with upper respiratory infections, acute alimentary upsets causing diarrhoea and vomiting, various indefinite aches and pains, worries about family, job, or health, and general malaise masquerading in various ways. And if a prescription is appropriate it is usually for an analgesic, and then instead of a prescription the patient can reasonably be told to take a couple of aspirins when the pain is bad.

GPs vary enormously in the number and kind of prescriptions they give, the number and kind of investigations they order and the proportion of patients whom they refer for a consultant's opinion.

The prescribing costs of the average GP are about £30 000 per annum. GPs may admit that many of their prescriptions are unnecessary, but excuse themselves on the ground that patients expect a prescription and it takes too long to argue them out of bad habits. But some succeed. The prescription costs of Ryde[5] (1976), who works in a SE London suburb among patients largely of social classes IV and V, are about 20% of average. He comments that as an assistant he 'was instructed by several principals to conclude every consultation with a prescription, to avoid complaints'. He believes there is a strong case against placebos and that a doctor's prescribing costs are inversely proportional to his grasp of the problem and his understanding of the patient and points out that medicine and tablets for a cold can suggest a repeat visit for every such incident through the years. And he asks: 'Is there evidence that a patient is in any way better off for taking cough medicines, laxatives, anorectics, lozenges, diarrhoea mixtures or gargles? Is there one psychoactive drug to remove psychological symptoms? If there were, no-one need by anxious again'. Ryde prescribes antibiotics, digoxin, diuretics, hormones, anxiolytics, analgesics, antacids and antihistamines, but only one third as frequently as the average GP.

Marsh[6] (1977) and his partners, along with health visitors and nurses, educated patients about minor illness, urged them to buy their own cough mixtures, diarrhoea mixtures, headache tablets etc. and encouraged self-reliance. In this way they achieved far more than any of the team members expected in a comparatively short time and reduced the number of prescriptions in the partnership by 19% compared to the previous year.

In the long run there are good grounds for saying that anorectics do more harm than good and there is no evidence that they help people to sustain marked weight loss indefinitely. If the peripheral vasodilators were abolished altogether mankind would be unharmed, apart perhaps from a few people with the Raynaud phenomenon. No preparation can justifiably be called a tonic. Clear-cut indications for prescribing antibiotics are uncommon. Very few people are deficient in vitamins. If diarrhoea and cough mixtures have any effect at all, this is very small. Yet all these groups of drugs are prescribed on an enormous scale. It is possible to argue that in some situations it is safer to prescribe antibiotics than not to prescribe them, but this excuse is rarely applicable to the other groups of drugs. Cyanacobalamin is widely prescribed as a 'tonic' and also for patients with multiple sclerosis and other diseases of the nervous system, but there is absolutely no evidence that it does good. Many non-anaemic patients are prescribed iron and many obese people are prescribed thyroxin.

The most frequently prescribed group of drugs are the psychotropics. In 1979 there were 44 million prescriptions of these in England, with a population of 46 million. No doubt there are good grounds for some of these prescriptions and it is impossible to lay down criteria to indicate when they should be used. Nevertheless, can anyone doubt that 44 million prescriptions is grossly excessive? The reason for many prescriptions is insomnia. In elderly people hypnotics may perhaps be justified sometimes, but when a doctor first prescribes hypnotics for a young person he should search his conscience. For when the patient has taken these for a time, he is likely to carry on with them indefinitely. Digoxin is valuable to patients with rapid atrial fibrillation, but it is prescribed on a huge scale to patients in normal sinus rhythm who have, or were thought to have in the past, cardiac failure, and here its value is most uncertain.

Doctors are constantly bombarded with circulars from the DHSS urging them to use the official names, rather than the proprietary names, of drugs when prescribing, as this is usually much cheaper. These circulars also give lists of groups of drugs with similar action and the cost of the most expensive may be many times greater than the cheapest. Many doctors nevertheless habitually prescribe proprietary and expensive drugs.

The total cost of NHS prescribing in general practice in Britain is about £500 million per year. And each inhabitant has on average six prescriptions from his GP per year. If all GPs prescribed along the same lines as does Ryde[6], the cost would fall to £100 million per year. Can anyone doubt that the populace would in consequence be far better off? GPs themselves would have more satisfactory lives, because they would have convinced their patients that colds, diarrhoea and other minor upsets get better irrespective of treatment and that, for relieving minor pain, aspirin is just as effective as the doctor's prescriptions. People would not, therefore, attend the surgery so often with these trivial maladies. GPs would have more time to listen to the problems of unhappy and worried people who are too often just given a prescription for a psychotropic drug.

REFERRAL TO HOSPITAL

The number of patients referred to hospital by GPs has been steadily rising for years. At present about 16% of the population are referred each year to out-patient departments as new cases. In addition, 20% of the population attend casualty departments, many of whom are referred by GPs. There is an enormous difference between GPs in the numbers referred, ranging from 20 per 1000 patients per year to over 250 per 1000. Fry[7] (1977) reduced his referral rate in 25 years from 105 per 1000 patients to 47 per 1000. He attributed this to greater experience and knowledge of the natural history of common disease and greater awareness of the limitations of consultants.

A clear indication for referral is that the GP believes an operation should be considered. On the other hand, if the patient and relatives suggest the possibility of an operation and the GP does not think this would help he can rightly say so and not refer the patient to a surgeon. This is particularly relevant to those operations for which there are no firm indications, such as tonsillectomy in children. The GP can of course be in error for referring patients too little. If a young man with a hernia is told to get a truss he can be severely condemned.

Perhaps the second strongest indication for referral is abnormal bleeding. The GP cannot properly deal with most patients with haemoptysis, haematemesis, melaena or passing blood per rectum, haematuria, or intermenstrual bleeding. Even here there may well be reasons for not referring. If an advanced chronic bronchitic has a haemoptysis, the kindest plan will probably be to keep him away from hospital, since whatever is amiss there is no possibility of useful treatment and therefore no point in doing investigations. And if a man who is known to have a duodenal ulcer passes a black stool there is no reasonable doubt as to the cause of the bleeding and, if he has clearly not lost much blood, he can rightly be kept at home.

In other than these two situations it is impossible to lay down any kind of criteria to indicate which findings justify referral and every GP must make up his own mind. Perhaps the one guiding principle should be that there is a possibility that the patient will benefit by referral.

In practice, an important reason why patients are referred is that they, or their relatives, request or 'demand' a specialist's opinion. Some GPs invariably yield to the slightest suggestion that a specialist might help, and there is apparently a common belief among the public that everyone has a 'right' to a specialist's attention. This matter is discussed from another angle in Chapter 7, p. 122. There I conclude that people do not have a 'right' to see a specialist and that if a GP believes that referral is futile, he should say so. Indeed, the GP can often benefit his patients by refusing to refer them, as they may be saved from pointless investigations and futile operations. The only right that patients have if they dislike the advice of their GP is to change him. Of course in practice every GP must be influenced by the desires of patients and relatives about referral. When an unfortunate patient has some unpleasant malady for which nothing useful can be done, it may still be reasonable to refer him just to convince him and his relatives that everything possible has been done.

Many referred patients, especially those seen by physicians, are emotionally disturbed people with psychosomatic symptoms. I estimated[8] (Todd, 1978) that at least one third of the patients referred to me came into this category, and there was a large psychological element in many others. Indeed, among patients with long-standing malaise, the severity and often the nature of the symptoms is partly determined by the emotional state, even though there is also some gross organic lesion. I used to feel that analysing symptoms, attempting to determine the extent to which they were emotionally caused and inquiring into the patient's fears about his health were of great help in management, as well as being most interesting to me. For at least sometimes this approach enabled reassurance to be given which appeared to help. But many physicians make little attempt to delve into the psyche; they consider themselves to be experts in some system, in which they diagnose, or endeavour to exclude, organic disease. And when they meet a patient who is evidently introspective and worried, with manifest psychosomatic symptoms, they perhaps brush him aside as just another neurotic or as having a large 'functional overlay'. In an obituary letter[9] to the *British Medical Journal* (1978) about D. Evan Bedford, perhaps the most celebrated British cardiologist of his time, appeared this passage: 'Bedford's appearance was not immediately striking, but was nevertheless memorable: the old tortoiseshell glasses, the inevitable cigarette left smouldering in the corner of his mouth, the raised eyebrows and wrinkled forehead while he considered a suitable reply to a question on a controversial subject and the languid and injured expression when he found himself confronted by a patient whose history exhibited a large element of neurosis'.

In Chapter 7, p. 118 I advance the view that all clinicians should be generalists much of the time, especially when dealing with patients who are persistently unwell. I also conclude that the supreme generalist should be the GP and that so many patients present a general problem. The GP should be the most suitable person to deal with patients of this kind, and often they derive nothing but harm from being referred to hospital, where they have futile investigations and never see anyone who looks at them as people. Unfortunately, even some GPs fail to take this general approach; like so many committed specialists they too look at patients not as people but as aggregations of organs.

Hopkins (1976) estimated[10] that each neurologist sees on average one new case of multiple sclerosis each month, yet this is said to be a common - if not the commonest - neurological disease. In the same period he will see about 100 patients with non-specific headache or migraine. How can a neurologist do better with headache patients than can a GP? No doubt many of these patients are referred as 'query cerebral tumour' and some have exhaustive investigations. Yet any doctor can conclude that most long-standing continuous or recurrent headache is not due to a cerebral tumour if he will only sit back and look at the whole patient against his background. The GP should be able to do this better than any consultant, because of his personal knowledge of the patient.

Apart from patients who are thought to need operations, patients referred for help with management rather than diagnosis include many dermatological problems, diabetics, the obese, hypertensives, asthmatics, and some subjects of the rheumatic diseases. Because of the NHS regulations, referral is necessary sometimes to obtain certain appliances; only a consultant can sign a form for a wheel chair. In addition, there are such highly specialized units as infertility and psycho-sexual clinics where both investigation and treatment are given.

INVESTIGATIONS

For many years the number of investigations has been increasing exponentially. In the NHS pathological tests have been doubling every 7 years and X-rays doubling every 12 years. The rate of increase is only dropping slowly. New investigations are constantly being introduced, many complicated and expensive. A machine for computer assisted tomography, about the spectacular success of which we have recently heard so much, costs around £250 000.

In the United States especially, but to a growing extent in Britain and other countries, investigations are being done as part of the regular health check which has become so popular among the upper echelons of the business world. And the number of investigations done at each attendance has steadily increased, especially since the development of the multi-channel analyser. This matter was considered in Chapter 4, p. 56, where the conclusion was reached that all this activity is almost wholly futile and liable to do more harm than good. The cost of it all is enormous, but in Britain this does not fall on the NHS.

In the United States many patients who attend hospital have various routine investigations. To a variable extent this happens in Britain. In chest clinics, for example, patients often have a chest X-ray at each visit to the hospital, before they see the physician. This 'saves' time as he can then see the X-ray picture while he is examining the patient.

When patients are admitted to hospital they are more likely to have some routine investigation. All patients who are to have an operation are liable to have a chest X-ray and, if above a certain age, an e.c.g., perhaps at the insistence of the anaesthetist. They may also have a haemoglobin and perhaps other pathological tests. Some physicians regularly do numerous investigations on all their in-patients so as to obtain a 'profile'. All this activity is costly; does it provide any safeguard or benefit the patient?

Korvin and others (1975) analysed[11] the records of 1000 patients admitted to a Vancouver hospital, each of whom had 20 chemical and haematological tests. 2200 of these tests were deemed abnormal and yielded 83 new diagnoses, but in no single case did a patient derive unequivocal benefit. The solitary patient who might have benefited was thought possibly susceptible to liver damage from halothane anaesthesia, and even this was uncertain. Possible benefit to one person from 20 000 tests is, in the authors' words, 'not impressive'.

There is, then, no justification for doing routine investigations on every in-patient. No doubt, it is reasonable to X-ray chests pre-operatively when patients have a cough or are breathless, but it is absurd to do so in the absence of symptoms, especially in the young. To do routine investigations on all out-patients is even more absurd.

A common reason why many investigations are done is to exclude a particular disease. When in fact the investigation does so, it may be most useful. But commonly the requested investigation will not exclude the disease in question. A normal e.c.g. does not exclude coronary artery disease, a normal e.e.g. excludes nothing, a normal barium meal does not exclude duodenal ulcer, a normal chest X-ray does not exclude carcinoma bronchus and normal bone X-rays do not exclude osseous metastases. Similar examples could be multiplied indefinitely.

Some physicians may do a vast series of investigations in an attempt to exclude every conceivable organic disease. The basis for this lies in the doctrine that, before a patient is decreed neurotic, every possibility of organic disease must be excluded. This doctrine was widely accepted a few decades ago and is still alive today among the mechanistically minded who ignore the patient and concentrate the attention on his organs. Among all the mistaken doctrines swallowed by the medical profession, this is one of the most absurd. The only reason for saying that someone is neurotic is that he is neurotic, and that conclusion is reached by talking to him and looking at him as a person. He may or may not have organic disease in addition to his neurosis. A result of this doctrine was that numerous patients who had psychosomatic symptoms were given such absurd 'organic' diagnoses as visceroptosis, hyperchlorhydria, sinusitis, chronic·gastritis, and diverticulitis because of the finding of irrelevant abnormalities in the process of 'excluding organic disease'.

Goldberg (1977), a consultant radiologist, entitled his article[12] 'Department of Inappropriate Investigations'. Among his conclusions were that the largest single group of X-ray requests came from the casualty department. A common excuse for the casualty X-rays is that if they are not taken there will be medicolegal complications (in spite of the fact that no British Court has found a doctor negligent for not taking an X-ray when, after properly examining the patient, he reached the decision that an X-ray was unnecessary; this is not so in the United States). Fewer than 1% of casualty skull X-rays revealed fractures. Many casualty officers order X-rays before they see the patient. Among irrelevant out-patient investigations Goldberg mentions X-rays of the neck and back in patients over 50 for backache and neckache, since abnormalities are usually found which in no way help to explain the symptoms. The occupants of coronary care units are liable to have daily, or even twice daily chest X-rays. Urgent barium meal or enema X-rays are requested in very ill aged patients, apparently in case the relatives refuse postmortem permission. Patients who are known to have widespread secondary deposits may have barium meal and follow through, barium enema, intravenous pyelography and liver and bone isotope scans.

Burns-Cox (1979), a consultant physician, asks the following questions[13]: 'Is there any evidence that bacteriological tests on the sputum of the chronic bronchitic with an acute chest infection are helpful? Is there any evidence that measuring the blood fats in adults has ever been of use to a single patient? How often do (plasma levels of urea and electrolytes) which are requested routinely on a high proportion of patients, affect the care of the patient? Is there any evidence that a routine chest X-ray in patients with presumptive cardiac infarction is necessary?' He comments: 'the multiple measuring haematology machine is a menace and nearly as harmful as the biochemical multichannel measurer; the routine measurement of serum iron and iron-binding capacity is a sure sign that the doctor emanates from an institution where measurements are worshipped at the expense of common sense; as soon as a laboratory (for pulmonary function tests) is opened, all of a sudden anaesthetists and other clinicians find themselves unable to carry on without the "reassurance" of these tests'.

Whenever a patient has glycosuria some doctors order a glucose tolerance test almost as a reflex action. This is very rarely needed to determine whether or not the patient has diabetes. If there is thirst and polyuria along with glycosuria, the symptoms alone make the diagnosis certain. If there is symptomless glycosuria a single elevated blood sugar is sufficient. The test is time-consuming and involves repeated venepuncture. (A patient once aptly remarked that he had had a glucose endurance test.) It is apparently done because it is thought to be 'scientific', providing documentary evidence both of the existence and severity of diabetes. This is absurd. The severity of diabetes is best assessed by the symptoms. Moreover, the obese maturity onset diabetic, the commonest type, may have a grossly abnormal glucose tolerance test when first diagnosed, but if he restricts his diet sufficiently may later have a near-normal, or even quite normal, curve.

Perhaps the most useless of all common investigations is the electroencephelogram. Whenever a patient is reported to have had a 'blackout' or other disturbance of consciousness an e.e.g. may be requested automatically. The common question we wish to have answered here is: did the patient have a faint or a fit? The e.e.g. cannot give the answer. Most epileptics have a normal e.e.g. between attacks. And if the e.e.g. is of a type which often accompanies epilepsy, this cannot prove that the patient had a fit. The main way of deciding between fit and faint is from a description by the bystanders of what happened. If this is equivocal, no investigation will give an unequivocal answer. If it is certain that the patient had a fit, we wish to know whether this was idiopathic or symptomatic. Here, the e.e.g. may sometimes hint that there is a space-occupying lesion, though more often it does not help to make this distinction.

A few decades ago the electrocardiogram was greatly overvalued as an indicator of coronary artery disease. Eminent cardiologists then stated that a repeatedly normal e.c.g. excluded cardiac infarction. This is now generally accepted to be absurd. In addition, undoubted angina of effort can be accompanied by a normal resting or even post-exercise e.c.g. Because of the imperfections of the e.c.g. coronary arteriography is widely practised in some advanced circles as a means of investigating precordial pain. This is totally unjustified. Coronary arteriography is risky and expensive and the only good reason for performing it is that a patient has symptoms of such severity that coronary bypass surgery is a possibility. In the two years before I retired I did not see one such patient, though many people with coronary artery disease were under my care.

As soon as some new diagnostic machine appears on the market, there is a rush to use it. To some extent this is justified, since the value of a machine can only be assessed by using it. Nevertheless, as a rule there is not much delay before the value of the machine and the indications for using it become clear. Perhaps the machine which has made the greatest impact recently is computer-assisted tomography. As a means of elucidating some CNS problems it is clearly a great advance. It will usually distinguish between cerebral haemorrhage, cerebral infarction, glioma, and metastasis. But as a rule this is of little consequence since whichever condition is present there is no useful treatment (except very occasionally for glioma). Only when there is a possibility of a remediable lesion, such as an extradural or subdural haematoma, abscess, or meningioma does the procedure help to determine the treatment. As soon as computer-assisted tomography became available in the hospital to which I referred patients for possible craniotomy I consciously sought suitable patients. In the 2 years before retiring I did not find a single one.

Thyrotoxicosis is often one of the easiest of all diagnoses to reach; even a brief glance from a distance is enough. But as each new investigation has been introduced — basal metabolic rate, serum cholesterol, protein-bound iodine, radio-iodine uptake, serum thyroxin, serum tri-iodothyronine, thyroid stimulating hormone etc. — many physicians invariably use them in these obvious cases. There is no possible advantage in this. No test assesses the severity of the condition nearly as well as does the clinical picture. And the common practice of doing repeated tests to assess the response to treatment is futile.

The only sound reason for doing thyroid function tests is when there is clinical uncertainty as to whether the patient is hyperthyroid. Here, many physicians believe there is clinical uncertainty when if they would only sit back and look at the patient as a whole it would be evident that she is not thyrotoxic. The nervous young woman with a poor appetite, cold extremities, trembling and tachycardia who complains of sweaty hands is not thyrotoxic, though is often wrongly thought to be so. If she is on the Pill and is found to have raised protein-bound iodine this has been taken as 'proof' of the diagnosis, which is an appalling error. There are of course genuinely doubtful cases, especially among the old. Here the assumption tends to be made that some test really does give a Yes or No answer to the question: Is the patient hyperthyroid? There is no reason to make this assumption. In any case, when the clinical picture is equivocal, the thyroid function tests tend to be equivocal.

There is an element of 'keeping up with the Joneses' when sophisticated diagnostic machines are introduced. Those in the hospitals which have not been allotted a new machine are liable to feel deprived and may talk of the inevitable 'lowering of standards' unless they can have one. And an appeal may be made to some rich tycoon or to the public to provide the machine which the parsimonious DHSS says it cannot afford. We are told that when computer-assisted tomography became available in the United States hospital after hospital ordered machines until President Carter put restrictions upon their import.

We doctors, then, overinvestigate on a colossal scale, wasting the patient's time and the nation's wealth in the process. The prime way of stopping this waste is for each doctor to ask himself when considering each investigation: 'Whatever the result of the investigation, will it alter my opinion?'. If the answer is No, the investigation should not be done.

FOLLOW-UP OUT-PATIENTS

GPs are responsible for new out-patients; consultants decide whether or not they should be followed up. Loudon (1976) noted[14] that in 1973 each consultant general physician and his junior staff dealt with on average 12.1 new out-patients per week and 54.6 'old' patients (based on whole time equivalents). Each surgeon saw 22.2 new and 53.4 'old' patients.

The physician who has been referred a difficult diagnostic problem may naturally wish to see the patient again, usually after doing some investigations, and perhaps several times. But in most hospitals and most specialties many old out-patients are seen by a registrar or clinical assistant, and when such patients have been attending regularly they are rarely discharged. Moreover, when patients attend at infrequent intervals they often see a different junior doctor on each occasion. Many diabetics who had previously attended clinics in other hospitals told me that they never saw the same doctor twice. In many hospitals there is a custom to make an out-patient appointment automatically when each in-patient is discharged. In consequence, wretched patients with some advanced disease may have a long ambulance journey to hospital and surgical patients who have had a straightforward operation such as appendicectomy may have an equally unnecessary journey. When discharging a patient I always told the ward sister whether or not he should have an out-patient appointment. In spite of this, patients were sometimes wrongly given appointments because someone had taken it for granted that every one who left hospital should attend out-patients.

When someone is attending a hospital indefinitely, the hospital doctor is taking the place of the GP. How often is this justified? If the consultant invariably sees the patient himself, he may be able to make the reasonable excuse that he is particularly interested in the patient, or in his malady, even though there is no other reason for attendance. But when the 'old' patient sees a succession of registrars this excuse does not hold. How often are there grounds for believing that the registrar has some expertise that the GP lacks, or that there is some other reason why the patient should remain under hospital care? It may be hinted in hospitals that many GPs are not to be trusted to carry out treatment properly, especially for, say, diabetics and hypertensives. No doubt there is truth in this sometimes, but the general assumption that hospital treatment is superior to GP treatment is ridiculous and the reverse may well be true. And if the standard of GP care is poor, the way to improve it is not to replace the GP by the hospital.

In spite of all this there may be grounds why certain patients should continue to attend hospital indefinitely. This is possibly true of diabetics on insulin, of some patients with malignant disease, and of patients attending fertility clinics and other highly specialized departments. And some patients may be involved in a research programme. But the main reason for many hospital attendances is not to benefit patients but to provide employment for registrars. Registrars rarely have any inducement to discharge patients. One can hardly imagine two registrars discharging nearly all the patients whom they had inherited from their predecessors and then informing their chief that they have so diminished their workload that one of them will not be needed in future. On the contrary, they will more likely complain that their workload has become intolerable, and their chief will make strenuous efforts to increase the establishment by another registrar in order to maintain 'standards'.

Loudon (1976) comments[14]:, 'It is remarkably difficult to alter the situation. Perhaps GPs should cancel unnecessary follow-up appointments ... I do so fairly often and invariably the consultant replies that he agrees, sometimes adding that he finds it impossible to stop "the system".'

The number of 'old' out-patients could be reduced to a fraction of the present figure with nothing but benefit to suffering humanity. The main responsibility for this state of affairs must be placed upon the consultants.

UNNECESSARY ADMISSIONS

A large proportion of all health resources are devoted to 'acute' in-patients. They are the most expensive users of the NHS, the cost per patient per week being over £300. They consume the most expensive features, such as high technology equipment in the operating theatre and the intensive treatment unit. Each unnecessary admission, therefore, wastes a great deal of money.

Surgery

The surest means of avoiding unnecessary admissions to a surgical ward is by not doing an operation. No-one disputes that in the past many operations were done without good reason. Surgeons pleated stomachs to cure gastroptosis, opened skulls to allow the brains of microcephalics to enlarge, fixed kidneys to cure nephroptosis, performed gastro-jejunostomies to cure duodenal ulcer, removed colons to cure intestinal auto-intoxication,and shortened the round ligaments to cure backache 'caused' by a retroverted uterus.

Perhaps the common operation for which the indications are most doubtful is tonsillectomy. There is more than a 50-fold difference in its incidence between different parts of the country. A medical student told me that a GP who examined him when he joined his medical school remarked that he could distinguish between doctor's children and others by looking at their throats: the tonsils of the doctor's children were still there but the tonsils of the others were missing. If tonsillectomy in children ceased altogether there is no evidence that anyone beyond that tiny number with mechanical obstruction would suffer, whereas every year a few children die after the operation, others have unpleasant complications, and perhaps many are upset emotionally.

Most patients with persistent abdominal symptoms cannot be given a pathological diagnosis, and the longer the symptoms have been present and the greater their number, the less is the likelihood that a pathological diagnosis can be made. Exasperated by the complaints of such patients it is all too easy to operate and remove, say, a 'chronic appendix' or a gallbladder which, even if it contains stones, has no connection with the symptoms.

In middle-aged women a popular operation is hysterectomy. If the patient has much bleeding and discomfort this can be most satisfactory. But it is widely believed that hysterectomy is commonly advised on insufficient grounds. To some extent this can be attributed to 'demands' by menopausal women that their uteruses are removed, but this does not excuse a surgeon who gives way to these 'demands' without good reason. On the other hand, it is said in some feminist circles that doctors are too eager to advise hysterectomy for heavy menopausal bleeding. Thus, 'Some doctors attempt to "solve" the bleeding problem by performing a hysterectomy. There are other, less drastic forms of treatment' (Phillips and Rakusen, 1978)[15].

Many operations are done for cosmetic reasons. And some, such as the removal of ugly facial scars, can be profoundly beneficial. But when the only criterion is appearance and the only reason for operation is pressure from the patient, it is easy to operate unwisely. Some women pay large sums for facelift operations or procedures to change the shape of their noses. In the short term the patients may be satisfied with the change in their appearance, but this satisfaction does not always persist. Perhaps the surgeon who persuades patients not to have operations of this kind will, in the end, do them the greatest service. Probably the commonest operations done mainly for cosmetic reasons are the varicose vein procedures. If ugly lumps can be made to disappear these may give lasting satisfaction. But the result is not always so satisfactory. The reason women ask for varicose vein operations is often to relieve the aching in their legs which they attribute to their veins. Unfortunately, some surgeons accept this theory. In fact, the aching appears to be related to the woman's awareness of the appearance of her legs. Men, who don trousers on rising and never give a thought to their varicose veins, rarely complain of aching.

Many operations for malignant diseases are palliative. A colostomy may be done for irremovable carcinoma of rectum, a cholecystenterostomy for carcinoma of the head of the pancreas, or a gastrectomy for carcinoma stomach or a lobectomy for carcinoma bronchus when there are already metastases. This is one of the most difficult areas in medicine, but one may suspect that too many such operations are done, especially in frail old people. The kindest course is often to leave well alone and give analgesics.

A recently devised operation now done on an enormous scale in America and a large and increasing scale in Britain is coronary bypass surgery. It has been claimed that when the left main artery is diseased this can actually prolong life, but it is too early yet to reach a firm conclusion. Otherwise, there is no evidence that it prolongs life and the justification for doing it is to relieve 'intractable' angina. For many years before retirement I only saw one patient who, after weight reduction and optimum doses of beta-blockers and trinitrin, seemed bad enough for coronary bypass surgery, though I saw many patients with angina. Yet some physicians refer large numbers of patients for surgery, and I suspect that far too many operations are done.

A recent trend has been to do many operations without admission on a day-bed basis. Hernia repair, varicose vein procedures, and termination of pregnancy are all widely performed in this way. But many surgeons have been reluctant to do this and, in their conservatism, look for reasons for insisting that the patient is always admitted and kept in for a week or more. Numerous papers have demonstrated the safety and patient satisfaction of out-patient surgery. If all surgeons did as many operations in this way as do the enthusiasts, there would be an enormous saving in bed occupancy.

Medicine

Many physicians, especially in teaching hospitals, regularly inform out-patients that they should be admitted for investigation or occasionally for treatment, so they are put on a waiting list. Perhaps weeks later they walk in carrying a suitcase. On the face of it, to admit such a patient into an 'acute' bed, of which we often hear we are so short, seems extraordinary. Is this ever justified?

Throughout my consultant career I never admitted a walking patient to an acute medical ward. The only patients I admitted from the out-patient department were acutely ill people who had been sent to out-patients by ambulance and were admitted immediately. A favourite dictum of mine was that if you can walk into a medical ward you needn't come in. All the investigations I ever thought desirable, including sigmoidoscopy, gastroscopy, barium enema X-rays, marrow puncture, and jejunal biopsy, could all be done in at most a few hours stay in the Day Bed Unit and very few needed that. Why, then, do so many physicians admit walking cases for investigation? Perhaps some complicated metabolic studies, cardiac catheterization and coronary arteriography justify admission. But the number of patients who are helped by metabolic studies is microscopic and the only legitimate grounds for cardiac catheterization and coronary arteriography is the possibility of surgery. The main basis for admission for investigation seems to be the persistence of bad habits acquired in the teaching hospital. The student is brought up with the idea that such admission is sound practice, so when he becomes a physician he carries on in the same way. And, when faced by a complicated problem in the out-patient department, instead of concentrating his mind and coming to a decision, he shelves the issue by saying 'you had better come into hospital for tests'. If it could only become accepted that admission for investigation is a badge of failure, as well as being distressing to the patient and wasteful of money, this regrettable practice would almost disappear.

Among the walking patients who are regularly admitted by some physicians for treatment are newly diagnosed diabetics for so called 'stabilization'. I have long maintained[16] (Todd, 1972) (see Chapter 7, p. 123) that the very concept of 'initial stabilization' is an absurdity, since when diabetics are first started on insulin they are not stable.

Obese people are sometimes admitted for months to be starved, only to put back the lost weight in the following months or years. Peptic ulcer subjects are, or at least recently were, admitted to medical wards for really 'energetic' treatment, though cimetidine has presumably made this less common. If peptic ulcer patients are getting such severe symptoms as to warrant admission the right course is, as a rule, to admit them for surgery. Aplastic anaemia needing repeated transfusions may be thought to justify the admission of a walking patient for treatment. I had 7 or 8 such patients over the years. I regularly saw them in the out-patient department one day, ordered a blood count and cross-match, arranged for them to attend the Day Bed Unit early on another day, a Saturday if they were at work, transfused them with four or so units of packed cells and sent them home again a few hours later.

EMERGENCY ADMISSIONS

Apart from the very few patients admitted immediately from the out-patient department, the responsibility for acute admissions rests mainly go the GP or the casualty officer. Patients who suddenly become unwell, or their relatives, have increasingly tended, especially during the small hours, to dial 999 for an ambulance rather than get in touch with the GP. They are then brought to hospital and usually admitted. When patients are asked why they did this they have sometimes replied that they did not like to get their poor overworked GP out of bed, especially as they 'knew' that at the hospital a doctor would be sitting there waiting for their arrival. Many such patients are discharged home later the same day.

There is no easy way of preventing unnecessary admissions due to dialling 999 for an ambulance. Casualty officers may sometimes admit people with minor injuries because of the fear of medicolegal consequences if they are sent home and later something goes wrong. But if the patient is properly examined, has a good home and it seems unlikely that anything grave has occurred, the casualty officer will hardly ever be successfully sued, even if some disaster does occur. Many casualty officers also too easily admit people who have taken overdoses of drugs, although they are fully conscious and seem well. This too may be for medicolegal reasons or because of the recommendation from the DHSS that all such patients should be seen by a psychiatrist. Fortunately, many such patients refuse to come in.

GPs vary widely in their admission policies. A common reason for emergency admission is sudden chest pain, which may be due to cardiac infarction. There has been an endless debate on this matter for years, and various studies have failed to show saving of life by admission. On the other hand, one strong ground for admission is the possibility of subsequent ventricular fibrillation, though the very act of moving the patient to hospital may make this more likely. If some hours have passed since the pain began and if the patient seems well and the pain has gone, the GP can properly advise in favour of remaining at home. Pain in the leg in a young woman (especially if she is on the Pill) is another common but questionable ground for admission. How bad should asthma or pneumonia be to justify admission? Much depends on the patient's circumstances, but many GPs too readily admit such people when they could reasonably remain at home.

UNNECESSARILY PROLONGED ADMISSION

We all agree that in the recent past many patients were kept in hospital needlessly long. Among them were young men who had had hernia operations, who remained in a hospital bed for perhaps 2 weeks, and those who had had cardiac infarcts, who often stayed for 6 weeks or more. Many patients are still kept in too long today.

In one common situation patients are detained because of the DHSS circular 'Hospital Treatment of Acute Poisoning' (1968). It is here recommended that in all cases of deliberate self-poisoning patients should be referred to designated treatment centres and seen by psychiatrists. When the NHS began one of the awful spectres dreamt up by its opponents was that ultimate horror of bureaucratic medicine, the issuing of edicts telling doctors how to treat their patients. This recommendation about self-poisoning is hardly an edict, yet in many hospitals all the physicians, instead of ignoring it, accept it as an edict and refer every single case of self-poisoning to a psychiatrist. This frequently results in the patient, who is perfectly well physically, remaining in hospital for several days. As there is no evidence that automatic psychiatric referral does good I invariably ignored this recommendation, deciding whether to retain or discharge patients according to the emotional state and circumstances of each one. Moreover, as Todd (1978) remarks[17]: 'Many junior doctors have an unfortunate antipathy towards their self-poisoning patients. It is my feeling that this is produced, or at least encouraged, by the automatic referral of patients to psychiatrists. As a result the medical staff fail to acquaint themselves with this group of patients despite the fact that they often stay on the wards for a number of days waiting to be seen by the psychiatrist'.[17]

Some surgeons, as well as admitting patients for operations which other surgeons would do on an out-patient basis, regularly keep post-operative patients in for a long time. They may make a rule that no patient should be discharged with stitches still in place, as if to do this contravenes some Divine Law.

Some physicians regularly detain patients for longer than do others. They may have a 'standard' stay for particular maladies or make a rule that no-one should leave hospital with a haemoglobin level below a certain figure. Worst of all, they may insist that they should personally discharge each patient although they only attend each ward once per week. There are so many variables here, the patient's age, personality, home circumstances and the severity of the illness, that it is absurd to lay down a standard length of stay. If the patient is recovering, is anxious to go home and has relatives to look after him it is often sensible to let him go and continue treatment at home only a very few days after coming in with, say, a cardiac infarct, pneumonia, or asthma.

OCCUPATIONAL HEALTH SERVICE FOR THE NHS

An Occupational Health Service began in some hospitals a few years ago. This was not due to any demand by the NHS staff. A service of this kind may have a useful function in such dangerous industries as mining, since those who work for the service may be able to reduce the hazards. In the NHS there are a few special hazards. The staff sometimes acquire infections from patients, and in mental hospitals they are occasionally attacked by patients. Those who work in pathological laboratories, especially in the field of microbiology, sometimes become ill because they are in contact with virulent organisms. And those who work in radiological departments are exposed to radiation, though with modern equipment and protective measures this is a very small hazard. Would the institution of an Occupational Health Service throughout the entire NHS lessen any of these hazards? No evidence has been advanced that it would do so. Nor is it easy to find any prima facie grounds why it should.

The occupational health physician can no doubt occupy his time in carrying out pre-employment medical examinations and in rejecting on medical grounds those he considers to be 'unfit'. And such examinations can be repeated at regular intervals. But, as was noted in Chapter 4, p. 64, there is no evidence that this kind of activity improves health. And there is never any justification for rejecting someone on medical grounds except when he is a hazard to patients or other staff, and in the NHS this is hardly conceivable. Of course, the physician can tell each person he sees that she should not smoke, should not let herself put on weight and should take regular hard exercise. He can also issue general propaganda on these matters in the hospital. But those who work in the NHS can hardly be unaware of these ways of maintaining health. For many years I examined all the nurses who were starting training in my hospitals and I told each one of the ill-effects of smoking. Those who were non-smokers nearly all continued in this sensible way but I was never once aware that I persuaded one of the smokers to stop.

The pressure to begin an Occupational Health Service is one more example of 'Keeping up with the Joneses'. Many large and profitable industries have them and therefore the NHS should have one.

A full-blown Occupational Health Service would add considerably to the already enormous cost of the NHS. The DHSS has recently been back-pedalling on this matter, occupational health is not being expanded, and doctors already appointed are not being made consultants. Whether this change of emphasis is due to the realization that an Occupational Health Service would bring no benefit or whether it is merely part of an economy drive is a matter for speculation. The pity is that the service was ever allowed to get off the ground and add to the already monstrous waste in the NHS.

TREATMENT INVOLVING HIGH TECHNOLOGY

All surgery involves technology. Most operating theatres have changed from being just rooms where surgery is carried out to specially designed places containing expensive air-conditioning equipment. Without doubt, this lessens both the infective hazard and the overheating hazard to the patient and increases the comfort and with it the efficiency of the surgeon and the theatre staff. Many recently developed and expensive machines, such as colonoscopes and laparascopes, have enabled surgeons to carry out useful operations which previously involved laparotomy. Whatever the cost of all this, there can be no questioning its benefits.

Anaesthetics hardly advanced between its beginning in the 1860s until the 1930s. Throughout all that time almost the only anaesthetics were nitrous oxide, chloroform and ether, given with the simplest equipment, or often no equipment beyond the famous 'rag and bottle'. Since then there has been a beneficial revolution. This has been due partly to the new anaesthetic agents and partly to the new machines which maintain breathing when the muscles are paralysed by curare-like drugs or when the thorax is opened. All this has been a great advance, expensive though it has been.

Perhaps the greatest triumphs of high technology surgery and anaesthetics have been in the repair of congenital heart disease. By means of assisted respiration, artificial cooling and extracorporeal circulation most of those with congenital heart lesions have been greatly improved and many have been 'cured'. In addition, many patients with rheumatic heart disease have been much improved by the highly satisfactory valvulotomy for mitral stenosis or the valve replacement procedures.

On the other hand, whenever some advanced new technique is developed, there is always a strong temptation to use it for less than sound reasons. One may suspect that some people with small ventricular septal defects unaccompanied by symptoms or cardiac enlargement and discovered by accident have been advised repair on the highly doubtful grounds that future disability, and in particular future bacterial endocarditis, will be prevented. At present a commonly performed cardiac operation, especially in the United States, is coronary bypass surgery. Although this may be justified sometimes, there are grounds for believing that it is recommended far too frequently (see p. 86).

High technology has made it possible to perform severely mutilating operations without killing the patient. Among these are pelvic evisceration and the removal of such large lengths of intestine that the patient is dependent thereafter on intravenous feeding. It is more than doubtful whether these are justified.

Intensive Treatment Units (ITUs) and Coronary Care Units (CCUs) have now become an accepted part of the hospital scene. They are vastly expensive both in terms of staff and of equipment costs.

The principle of putting the patients needing intensive care into one unit seems eminently sensible. It may even be thought to make economies possible, by concentrating the expensive equipment into one place and by lessening the number of staff in the ordinary wards. In practice, the possible economies are probably small or absent. The important practical question is 'How often does intensive care save lives which are worth saving?'. During my last 5 years before retirement I saw two medical patients only whose lives were undoubtedly saved by high technology treatment in an ITU. Both had respiratory paralysis accompanying Guillain-Barré syndrome and were treated by tracheostomy and assisted respiration. Both made complete recoveries. I saw one other patient whom we hoped would be saved by similar action. He had severe tetanus and was treated by curare-like drugs along with tracheostomy and assisted respiration, but he died of sudden pulmonary embolism. There were a few other patients, including severe asthmatics, the poisoned and those with diabetic ketosis, who recovered, but they would probably have recovered in an ordinary acute medical ward. And there were a few respiratory cripples whom we tided over an acute exacerbation, though whether we were taking the kindest action by so doing was indeed questionable.

Surgical patients are more likely to be helped by intensive care than are medical patients. Among them especially are those with severe chest injuries, who would die without assisted respiration. Those deeply unconscious after head injuries can also be kept alive by intensive care until they recover, though unfortunately a number never do recover appreciably and are kept alive living a vegetable existence indefinitely. After some operations too intensive care may help.

In practice patients for whom intensive care is appropriate are uncommon in the average hospital. But when there are no suitable patients the ITU is not usually kept empty; it is occupied by unsuitable patients, mainly those who are very ill but for whom little can be done. It can be argued that this is better than having the staff sitting around doing nothing, or transferring the staff temporarily to other wards (from whence they may have to be recalled in a hurry later).

A critical eye can be cast on many of the activities which commonly occur in ITUs. The monitoring devices are extremely expensive, both in outlay and, because they so often go wrong, in upkeep and one may doubt whether they often save lives. Blood gas analyses are often done repeatedly, but I hardly ever recall occasions when these gave significant help. One would see enormously high CO_2 levels in respiratory cripples, but the gravity of the situation was evident by glancing at the patient. Electrolytes are regularly estimated, perhaps many times daily. Sometimes this is possibly helpful, but too often it is not. There is always a strong tendency to 'correct' any abnormalities discovered by the intensive observations. If the blood pressure drops dopamine is given to raise it; if it is too high methyldopa or hydralazine are given to lower it. If the haemoglobin is below a certain level a blood transfusion is given; if it is above another level venesection is performed. If there is acidosis lactate or bicarbonate are given in the drip; if there is alkalosis, ammonium chloride is given instead. If the serum potassium is low, potassium chloride is added to the drip, if serum potassium is high, an ion exchange resin is given. If there are ectopic beats, lignocaine may be added to the drip; if there is 2:1 heart block atropine may be prescribed. All these things are done in the hope of saving life, but it is too easily taken for granted that 'correcting' some parameter will have this effect.

The one life-saving measure which takes place in CCUs is giving a DC shock for ventricular fibrillation. This can of course be given anywhere in the hospital, but there are clear advantages in concentrating all the patients likely to develop this arrhythmia in one place where a DC shock machine is available. Otherwise, the value of CCUs is most doubtful (as was noted above) and moving patients to hospital from their own beds may increase the likelihood of ventricular fibrillation. In so far as patients with definite or suspected cardiac infarction are admitted to hospital the sensible policy is to put them all in the CCU, however transient their pain. In practice, most patients in CCUs do not need intensive *care* (now that the appalling practice of keeping the patients at absolute rest is dead); they need intensive observation in case ventricular fibrillation develops. If a patient develops heart block causing unpleasant symptoms, pacing is clearly appropriate. Otherwise, the value of the activities common in CCUs - giving lignocaine to prevent extra-systoles, giving metaraminol or dopamine for cardiogenic shock, and pacing just because there is 2:1 block or even total block if it is symptomless - is unproven.

RADIOTHERAPY

Apart from surgery and intensive care, the main treatment involving high technology is radiotherapy. Associated with this is cancer chemotherapy, which may be used as an adjuvant or an alternative. These can be lifesaving for some victims of chorionepithelioma, Hodgkin's disease, carcinoma of uterus, and acute lymphatic leukaemia. And they can cause prolonged remissions with great symptomatic relief for patients with lymphosarcoma and other reticuloses. But only a minority of the patients given radiotherapy of chemotherapy have these favourable conditions; the majority are affected by such unpleasant maladies as cerebral glioma, carcinoma of the bronchus with or without overt metastases, and metastases from a variety of primary growths. Most of these unfortunate people derive neither significant increase in their span of life nor an improvement in the quality of life and they may suffer unpleasant side-effects.

Radiotherapy and cancer chemotherapy should only be given when there is a reasonable hope either of cure or of prolonged and marked improvement. This restraint is only likely to be achieved because patients are not referred to radiotherapy departments, not because radiotherapists refuse to prescribe treatment (see Chapter 7, p. 120).

PHYSIOTHERAPY, OCCUPATIONAL THERAPY, AND SPEECH THERAPY

Especially among 'rheumatic' patients there is great demand for physiotherapy. Indeed, when a patient has a painful part it may seem obvious that treatment should be applied directly to it. If physiotherapy is not prescribed, the patient may apply a domestic source of heat to the part, wrap it in cotton wool, or rub in embrocation.

If a doctor were to send a patient with a prescription for 'drugs' to the chemist he would rightly conclude that the doctor had taken leave of his senses. But many patients sent to physiotherapy departments are not prescribed any particular treatment; the request is made that physiotherapy - any kind of physiotherapy - be given.

There is no evidence that most kinds of physiotherapy do good. It is particularly used for maladies with a variable course and it is easy to attribute improvement to treatment which in fact is due to nature. There may also be a placebo effect which may well be more important with physiotherapy than with drugs. And double-blind clinical trials are impossible when assessing physiotherapy. Trials have been done in which alternate patients have been given some passive physiotherapy and alternate patients have been denied it. These have failed to provide convincing evidence of the value of the treatment.

There can nevertheless be no doubt of the value of some kinds of active physiotherapy. When a patient's muscles are weak exercises will strengthen them. Controlled trials are not needed to demonstrate that if a patient cannot walk properly he should practise walking. But exercise is self-treatment. The function of physiotherapists here is to tell patients what exercises to perform, to help them, and to provide apparatus. The hemiparetic who cannot walk unaided must be helped to become independent. When he is able to walk unaided improvement will be self-perpetuating.

Useful aids are provided in physiotherapy departments, such as the walking frame, which has a wide application. The badly affected rheumatoid arthritic may be helped to live independently by wearing specially made shoes for her misshapen feet, by devices to assist her to dress, and by gadgets to enable her to perform her chores. Other popular devices are of less certain value. Many patients wear back supports, sometimes for years. A patient may insist that provided she wears a special surgical corset her back pain is relieved and thereafter demands a new corset as the old one wears out. Should the doctor always give way to this demand? This is a difficult question. If she insists that without a corset she suffers agonies of pain the doctor can only allow her to have one. Nevertheless, if patients would only depend on their own muscles rather than supports one suspects that in the long run they would do better. Neck supports are popular for painful neck conditions. Although they are no doubt sometimes justified, one may suspect that they are used too much. Traction is widely used, especially to the pelvis for patients who are thought to have symptoms from lumbar disc lesions and to the neck for painful neck conditions. Sometimes it appears to be dramatically effective, but often it is not. Unfortunately, there do not seem to be criteria which indicate when, and what kind of, traction is likely to help.

Postural drainage and breathing exercises are advised for patients with respiratory conditions, and when they are acutely ill the physiotherapist tries to help them to bring up their secretions, by encouragement to cough, deep breathing, and percussion of the chest. Thereby it is hoped that the risk of lung collapse will be lessened. Whether or not this is generally effective it is impossible to say, though changes of posture and encouragement to move and cough may sometimes result in the expectoration of damaging plugs of sputum. Postural drainage for patients who have large amounts of sputum from bronchiectasis is without reasonable doubt helpful and by regularly lying in the appropriate posture much sputum can be got rid of. Here, the physiotherapists' function is to show the patient how best to drain himself. Thereafter the patient gives self-treatment. Asthmatics are advised to do breathing exercises, especially using their diaphragms, in the hope that these will better enable the patient to deal with the attacks. There is no clear evidence that such exercises are effective.

The benefits from physiotherapy are, then, small but the pressure on physiotherapy departments to provide 'treatment' is great. Much of this is due to patient demand. It can be argued that if a patient is determined to have physiotherapy he should have it, as otherwise he is likely to be resentful and blame his doctor for his persisting symptoms. No doubt this argument has some force, though no-one would apply it to most other remedies. The surgeon who removed an appendix because the patient demanded it would hardly excuse himself for so doing. The prime way of diminishing futile physiotherapy is by the development of a more critical attitude by doctors towards it. Moreover, passive physiotherapy by infra red, short wave, massage, etc. — the kind which patients especially 'demand' — is intrinsically unsatisfactory because it puts the onus of recovery upon the physiotherapist. Whereas active measures encourage the patient to recover by his own efforts.

Children who are born deaf can only be taught to speak by specialized techniques. Stammerers can be helped by other techniques. The treatment of both these categories is not the responsibility of the NHS. The adult patients who are given speech therapy in hospitals are mostly the victims of stroke or other cerebral disease.

The patient with dysphasia following a stroke usually improves with time, often strikingly. When dysphasia is persistent, speech therapy is often prescribed. Controlled studies of dysphasic people, in which alternate cases have been denied it, have not been made. There is, therefore, no firm evidence of the value of this treatment. But we can be sure that it has no dramatic effect, since many patients who are given it make little progress, and others who are not given it rapidly improve. The doctor is under the strongest pressure to do something for the dysphasic stroke victim. If he says that speech therapy is useless, the relatives and nurses may feel that just to do nothing is a counsel of despair. It may also be argued that the attention of the therapist may improve the patient's morale. In practice many stroke victims are given little or no speech therapy because of the paucity of therapists. But until unequivocal evidence of the value of speech therapy is advanced there can be no justification for increasing the number of therapists.

Occupational therapy is widely given to long-stay hospital patients as a 'diversionary' measure. Left to their own devices they may sink into boredom and apathy; if they are persuaded to occupy themselves in some useful way, by making something, they may be much happier. And sometimes this may actually aid recovery. But occupational therapists are apt to deride mere 'diversional' treatment as beneath them. It may be worth giving, but should be arranged, not by highly skilled occupational therapists, but by worthy volunteer ladies.

The hope is that occupational therapy has some specific effect in aiding recovery. The stroke victim with a partially paralysed arm seems a suitable subject. Without doubt using the arm increases the rate of improvement. But just performing a series of exercises over and over again may become so tedious that the patient gives up trying. If instead the occupational therapist devises some particular occupation which makes him use his affected hand he may carry on much longer. That this is beneficial can hardly be questioned, though the degree of benefit is probably small. In any case, occupational therapy is only appropriate for a few, and for the majority the most suitable occupation to aid recovery is their own occupation.

Occupational therapy has, then, a legitimate but small place. But it is given to many patients who are unlikely to be helped by it, except perhaps as a 'diversionary' measure. Indeed, this is probably the greatest benefit from occupational therapy, and it is a pity that some therapists take the view that 'diversional' treatment is beneath their attention.

THE VAST WASTE OF RESOURCES

In this chapter I have endeavoured to show how great is the waste in the NHS - waste for which doctors are almost wholly responsible. GPs hand out prescriptions costing £500 million per year, whereas their patients would be better off if this figure were reduced to one fifth or less. GPs admit to hospital many patients who could reasonably remain at home and they refer huge numbers to out-patients, many for no other reason than that the patients 'demanded' a specialist's opinion. Doctors of all kinds order investigations on a colossal scale, most of which could be avoided if investigations were only asked for if the result could influence the action taken. Surgeons do too many operations, they admit patients for operations which could be done without admission and they keep patients in hospital needlessly long. Physicians needlessly admit walking patients for investigation and sometimes for treatment and also keep patients in longer than necessary. A vast army of 'old' out-patients attend hospital, often indefinitely and usually seen only by junior doctors, for no good reason. Few patients benefit from the activities which characterize Intensive Treatment Units and the value of much of that activity is highly questionable. Far too much radiotherapy and cancer chemotherapy is given. Physiotherapy gives modest benefits to a few but it is prescribed on a huge scale for many.

Yet we doctors, instead of individually and collectively doing our best to abolish this monstrous waste, constantly complain that the NHS is falling apart because it is so underfinanced. And instead of blaming ourselves we blame the public demand, the politicians and the bureaucrats. Every prescription and every request for an investigation is signed by a doctor. Every patient's admission and every out-patient attendance is arrange by a doctor. If a surgeon does an unwise operation he alone should be blamed. If a radiotherapist orders unwise radiotherapy the fault is his.

In recent times one has hardly been able to open a medical journal without reading about the ever declining medical standards. If we would only prescribe less, refer less, investigate less, operate more wisely, give less radiotherapy and physiotherapy, admit less, and keep patients in hospital for less time nearly all our problems would be solved. And at the same time our standards of medical care would improve out of all recognition.

THE AWFUL PARADOX OF MEDICINE

One of the worst features of the medical scene in Britain today is the waiting lists. There may be a wait of many weeks to see a general surgeon and of many months to see an orthopaedic surgeon. After the surgeon has been seen and has advised an operation there may be a much longer wait for admission — up to 2 or 3 years in some districts. On the other hand, there are remarkable variations between different parts of the country and different hospitals. In some lucky places it is possible for a patient with a chronic condition to see a surgeon without delay and to be given an admission date in the near future. And if a patient has a condition which the GP thinks needs urgent attention, a surgeon can usually be seen with little delay and, if he advises operation, the patient is usually admitted with little further delay.

Although this situation is so deplorable, it is not quite so bad as it sounds. The waiting lists which we hear all about are the long ones; patients do not write to their MPs or threaten to sue the Secretary of State when they are admitted to hospital quickly. And some waiting lists provide no grounds for indignation. One of the longest waiting lists in many hospitals used to be for tonsillectomy in children. But as the reasons for doing this operation are so doubtful this delay is probably beneficial. When the child is finally sent for he may be no longer getting the frequent upper respiratory infections which were responsible for his referral to hospital, so the parents decline the proferred bed. But it is appalling that patients with, say, cataracts, painful osteoarthritic hips, hernias, and uterine prolapse causing persistent discomfort should have to suffer for years before having their operations.

A corollary of all this is that many people with innocent surgical conditions seek private treatment because they would have to wait for months or years before they could have operations under the NHS. Consequently, consultants have a vested interest in waiting lists; the longer they are the bigger their incomes are likely to be. Priority is given, not to those in the greatest need, but to those with the most money. This is the most unsavoury aspect of the matter. The individual consultant whose conscience cannot stand this situation has, of course, a simple remedy - to refuse to have private patients.

Thus, on the one hand we waste resources on an enormous scale, as described throughout this chapter. And, largely as a consequence of this, wretched patients with innocent surgical conditions have to wait indefinitely for relief. This is the awful paradox of medicine, and the blame for it rests almost entirely on the doctors. Patients may be stupid, politicians may make promises, and bureaucrats may be incompetent, but it is, to say the least of it, unbecoming of us doctors to be concerned with the motes in the eyes of our brothers before we have dealt with the beams in our own.

The often repeated claim that if only we spent more of the GNP on health the situation would be improved is absurd in the extreme. If all hospitals were given a lot more money this would probably be largely wasted on more high technology equipment and doctors would do even more useless investigations than they do at present.

Although we doctors have it in our collective power to transform the situation, certain individuals may be unable to solve their own problems, even though they are supremely wise. The individual orthopaedic surgeon may do no unnecessary investigations, may keep his patients in hospital for the shortest possible time, and only operate on those people whom he can, with reasonable certainty, benefit. But he may still find that more patients with, say, painful osteoarthritic hips who are evident candidates for total replacement are being referred to him than he can possibly deal with. What action can he take? First, he can reduce the numbers referred to him. He can do this either by writing to the local GPs to urge them not to refer patients without some compelling ground or by looking at all the GPs letters and selecting the most suitable cases. Second, he can ensure that he accepts for operation only that number of patients with which his team can deal, thus avoiding the development of a waiting list. This may involve his refusal to accept some patients who might be helped, but this is far better than keeping patients waiting for years when they undoubtedly would be helped. When dealing with most chronic surgical conditions there is a spectrum. At one end are patients for whom operation is clearly desirable, at the other end are patients who are unlikely to benefit from it, and in the middle are patients for whom the pros and cons are fairly evenly balanced. Some surgeons are 'conservative'. If all surgeons followed a more conservative line, most of these problems would be solved.

Although so many consultants — physicians, geriatricians and psychiatrists in particular — spend so much of their time in largely futile endeavour, orthopaedic surgeons may perhaps be a special case and their numbers should be increased. The reason for this can be largely attributed to the spectacular success of total hip replacement. Moreover, if a wholly satisfactory artificial knee joint can be devised, there will be a large back log of patients waiting for total knee replacement. But if only the existing orthopaedic surgeons would concentrate their attention on those patients they can most help, they could greatly improve the situation without an increase in their numbers. Surgeons who perform kidney transplants may be another special case, as there are so many suitable patients waiting for this. An important practical difficulty here is the shortage of cadaver kidneys. The simplest way of improving this situation would presumably be a change in the law to enable kidneys to be removed unless the dead person had left instructions that he did not wish to donate them. And if cyclosporin A fulfills its early promise, the reasons for doing kidney transplants will become much stronger.

SUMMARY

(1) There is a widespread but wrong belief that the deficiencies in the health service are due to a lack of resources.

(2) The only direct demand which the public can make on the NHS is to seek an interview with a GP or go to a casualty or VD department.

(3) GPs give far too many prescriptions and refer far too many patients to hospital.

(4) Many patients referred to hospital, especially to physicians, are emotionally disturbed and have psychosomatic symptoms.

(5) All clinicians should be generalists much of the time. GPs should be the supreme generalists.

(6) Far too many investigations are done. No investigations should be done as routine and many investigations will not exclude particular organic diseases.

(7) Far too many 'old' patients attend hospitals indefinitely.

(8) Too many operations are done. Many patients are admitted for operations which could be done a day bed basis.

(9) Walking patients should not be admitted to medical wards for investigation and very rarely for treatment.

(10) Many patients are needlessly admitted as emergencies, either by obtaining an ambulance and going direct to hospital or by their GPs.

(11) Many patients are kept in hospital for needlessly long periods.

(12) There is no evidence that an Occupational Health Service for the NHS is beneficial.

(13) Treatment involving High Technology is useful in a few specified situations, and especially for certain operations. But High Technology in Intensive Treatment Units and in other places has a very small application and is vastly overused.

(14) Far too much physiotherapy is prescribed. Occupational therapy and speech therapy have a very limited application.

(15) Although on the one hand resources are wasted on an enormous scale, there are long waiting lists for unfortunate patients needing operations for chronic conditions. This is the awful paradox of medicine and the responsibility for it rests almost wholly on the doctors.

References

1. Owen, D. (1976). *Lancet,* **1,** 1006
2. Ferriman, Annabel (1978). *Times,* 9 August.
3. Leading article (1974). *Br. Med. J.,* **1,** 247
4. Leading article (1977). *Br. Med. J.,* **1,** 792
5. Ryde, D. (1976). *Practitioner,* **216,** 557
6. Marsh, G.N. (1977). *Br. Med. J.,* **2,** 1267
7. Fry, J. (1977). *Proc. R. Soc. Med.,* **70,** 69
8. Todd, J.W. (1978). *Br. Med. J.,* **1,** 417
9. Obituary letter about D. Evan Bedford (1978). *Br. Med. J.,* **1,** 515
10. Hopkins, A. (1976). *Lancet,* **1,** 956
11. Korvin, C.C., Pearce, R.H. Stanley, J. (1975). *Ann. Intern. Med.,* **83,** 197
12. Goldberg, B.G. (1977). *Br. Med. J.,* **2,** 1274
13. Burns-Cox, C.J. (1979). *World Med.,* **14,** 84
14. Loudon, I.S.E. (1976). *Lancet,* **1,** 736
15. Phillips, A. Rakusen, J. (1978). *Our Bodies Ourselves. (London: Allen Lane)*
16. Todd, J.W. (1972). *J. R. Coll. Physicians,* **7,** 77
17. Todd, P.J. (1978). *Br. Med. J.,* **1,** 115

6

The Caring Side of the Health Service

In Chapter 5 I pointed out that the health services can be separated into the curing side and the caring side. When people talk of the 'infinite demands' on the NHS they are usually referring to the curing side. I reach the conclusion that much of the resources devoted to curing are wasted.

The caring side deals with all those unfortunate people who need an asylum because they cannot live independently in the community. Among them are the severely psychotic, the severely mentally subnormal and the senile geriatric. As the average age of the population rises more caring is needed. And there is already a general shortage of long-stay accommodation, with severe shortages in such places as the Sussex coast, where the proportion of old people is highest.

In practice, most care is provided, not by the NHS or the welfare services, but by relatives or neighbours. The most familiar of all care is that of parents for children. As a rule the burden steadily lightens as the children grow older, but if children are mentally defective, parents may devote their lives to them. When such a child has grown to be middle-aged perhaps one parent dies, leaving an even more awful burden to the other. Then in due course the remaining parent dies or becomes incapacitated, and suddenly for the first time a helpless mentally defective adult becomes the responsibility of the welfare authorities.

Otherwise, the commonest kind of care is that given by one spouse to another or by children to aged parents. When an ageing married couple are living alone sooner or later one usually begins to fail. The other may then take on the care of the failing one and be on duty for a 168-hour week with a never-ending chore, sometimes without a break for year after year. Unmarried daughters especially may devote years to the care of aged parents and in the end be left living an unhappy and lonely life in the family house.

Most surprising and touching of all can be the care of the old by neighbours. A kindly woman will naturally look in on an old neighbour upstairs or next door. In due course she may do some of the old person's shopping and then all of it. Next she perhaps takes on some or all of the cooking and washing and looks in many times daily. I have seen several examples of this, not as a doctor but as an ordinary citizen. The kindly person who acts like this may often grumble about the chore she has taken on but just hasn't the heart to insist that the old person is removed to a hospital or welfare home. And yet one often hears doctors complaining, or journalists writing, or clergymen preaching that people no longer bother with the old folks, as they did in the old days. No doubt many children and neighbours only take care of the old occasionally and unwillingly, or refuse altogether to help. There are no statistics on this matter, but my impression is that many people give quite a lot of care when the need arises.

The people who give this kind of care, so far from being paid for it, may actually lose money directly, as well as losing time (which, if they were not occupied in caring, they might well fill by doing a paid job). Of course the situation varies infinitely. Some old people who are looked after by neighbours insist on paying for these services. And a well to do old person living with relatives may contribute more to the family budget than he takes out. But if more financial inducements could be given many relatives or neighbours, who would otherwise insist that some old person must be removed to a hospital or home, would be more than willing to carry on in their caring role. This would be far less expensive than keeping the old person in an institution. Such an arrangement would involve administrative problems, as there would have to be criteria laying down the circumstances under which money is paid out. There would also have to be arrangements by which the old person could be temporarily put in hospital or home when the relatives or neighbours were on holiday. Another means of ameliorating the situation is the Day Hospital. A family still continues to look after an old person but is relieved of the burden during most of the daytime for 5 days every week.

When old people are living alone home helps and meals-on-wheels, perhaps along with visits by voluntary agencies, may help them to keep their independence. Valuable though these are, they are not of much use when help is most needed, that is when the old person is failing. There are still those long hours at night and longer hours at weekends when he has to manage by himself.

THE NEED FOR ASYLUM

An asylum was originally a sanctuary or refuge. In mediaeval times the hospitals under the auspices of religious orders were largely asylums for the frail and sick, who were cared for for the rest of their lives. By the 19th century the asylum had come to mean a lunatic asylum. Officially, we have had no lunatic asylums for many years; they have been replaced by mental hospitals. But the longterm inmates of these hospitals are still there because they cannot live in the outside world and need a protected asylum.

The other large category who need an asylum are the aged frail, and in particular the victims of senile dementia, who now occupy so high a proportion of the long-stay wards in the mental hospitals. Among the young, the severely mentally defective who are violent, uncontrollable and perhaps incontinent have an overwhelming need for an asylum. There are also a few tragic cases of young people with physical disability of such severity that they too need an asylum. Among them are quadriplegics after injury and the victims of advanced multiple sclerosis.

Some 250 000 people in Britain are in longterm hospital care, mostly in mental hospitals, geriatric wards, or hospitals for the mentally subnormal. (There are also many old people whose need is for an asylum but who are 'blocking acute beds' because they were admitted as emergencies, cannot be discharged home and are waiting a vacancy in a geriatric ward). Much of this accommodation is bad. Many mental hospitals are old and dingy. When a general hospital has old and new wards, the old wards are usually geriatric wards. Staffing ratios are much worse in longterm than in acute hospitals (no doubt rightly in some cases). Staff shortages are more likely, as most nurses and other staff prefer not to work with longterm patients. Less money is spent on food and various facilities than in acute hospitals. Yet a patient in an acute hospital is only there for a short time and if he has to submit to rules and privations he can look forward to a quick release. The asylum patient has to endure his lot indefinitely.

Many of the senile dements are so deteriorated that any pretence of rehabilitation is absurd. For all the other categories in longterm care the aim should be to encourage as much independence as possible. But in the words of Falck and Kane[1] (1971): 'It is in the nature of the institution that residents increase their dependency and tend to withdraw from meaningful involvement; but it is not inevitable that they do so. A strong awareness on the part of all staff is the minimum condition necessary to prevent the psychologically noxious aspects of life that occur in even the most luxuriously and physically active institution ... many institutions show strong tendencies to organize residents and activities so that the system runs efficiently from the standpoint of organization and administration. For example: ... insisting that all beds be made by 7 am ...; insisting that all residents get into their night clothes immediately after supper'.

In the hospitals for the mentally handicapped efforts have been made to reduce the dependency of the residents. Those in mental hospitals should be kept occupied throughout most of the day whenever practicable. And old people should be encouraged to do something, rather than to sink into boredom and apathy. The supreme practical difficulty in effecting these kinds of improvement is the cost involved.

A few decades ago there was a belief that if there were enough active geriatricians to ensure that old people had sufficient energetic treatment they would rarely become chronically sick, so there would only be a small need for long-stay geriatric beds. Especially after the introduction of psychotropic drugs, which improved the schizophrenics, there developed a similar belief that if there was sufficient activity by a sufficient number of energetic psychiatrists there would only be a small need for long-stay wards in mental hospitals. It became official DHSS policy that the large old mental hospitals should be phased out and that psychiatric services should be based on the district general hospitals. Both these beliefs were absurdly optimistic.

Geriatricians may admit that these considerations do not much apply to the senile dements, who are the largest category needing an asylum among the old. No doubt many old people can be helped to keep going by a variety of measures, such as appliances, remedial classes, better spectacles, and deaf aids. Most of the help needed does not involve doctors. The main principle behind these measures should be to encourage the old to keep, or to regain, their independence. And a most potent factor here is the character of the individual. 'The Lord helps those who help themselves.' But whatever is done we are likely in future to need increasing amounts of asylum accommodation for the old, because of the increasing average age of the population.

Many voices have been raised against the DHSS policy of phasing out the old longterm mental hospitals. Many occupants of these hospitals have also committed crimes and if they are discharged from the mental hospital to 'the community' they are liable to end up in prison. As Williams[2] (1979) points out, 'It appears that the Government's policy of phasing out psychiatric hospitals is playing a significant part in the build-up of mentally ill people in prison. The problem will continue unless adequate facilities for new long-stay patients are provided'. Bailey[3] (a visiting consultant psychiatrist to a prison and remand centre) comments (1979): 'A large number of mentally disordered offenders have a chronic condition and are often of no fixed abode, so they belong to no local authority or psychiatric hospital and no bed is available for them should a psychiatrist recommend their admission. More disturbed and violent offenders who might well be considered suitable for a special hospital under the DHSS cannot be admitted because of lack of accommodation . . .'

ALTERNATIVE KINDS OF ASYLUM

Although we need so much asylum accommodation, this must not necessarily be in hospital. One alternative asylum is prison, which is clearly inappropriate except for those who have committed some serious crime, if, indeed, it is appropriate for them when they are mentally disturbed. There are also hostels, hospices, reception centres, borstals and various types of old people's homes.

Many old people who had been living alone are admitted to hospital in emergency and never recover to the extent that they can be alone again. But they may well recover to the extent that they are suitable for a welfare home or even a flat where there is a resident warden. They nevertheless remain in hospital, if not 'blocking an acute bed' they are blocking a longterm bed, because there is a long waiting list for welfare homes. And when a vacancy does occur in a home priority may have to be given to some unfortunate person at the end of his tether living in his own home, rather than to the patient who is blocking a hospital bed. An important practical difficulty here is that hospitals are run by the DHSS whereas welfare homes are run by the local authorities. And anything which will put up the rates tends to be resisted. Yet welfare homes are less costly than hospitals. We can only hope that ways are found of overcoming this administrative situation and of encouraging the building of more welfare homes rather than long-stay geriatric wards.

The question constantly arises as to how 'fit' an old person has to be before he can go to a welfare home. The final decision may be left to the matron of the home and if she says someone is unsuitable, that is the end of the matter. In practice, people who are incontinent or need a great deal of help in looking after themselves are usually not admitted. On the other hand, when the inmates of welfare homes become incontinent, confused, or even bedfast, they may be allowed to remain there indefinitely. To lay down firm criteria distinguishing between the 'hospital case' and the 'welfare home case' is impossible, though futile attempts to do so have been made. In general, standards of admission to welfare homes have been set too high. One excuse for this is that there are so few staff that they are unable to clean up innumerable dirty beds, feed people, and help them in every activity. No doubt this is so, but the solution is to increase the staff rather than build more geriatric wards. Even the problem of incontinence, which looms so large, can be dealt with by indwelling catheters (for women) or perhaps by penile appliances (for men). These may result in urinary infection, but this is far better than keeping people permanently in hospital for no other reason than that they are incontinent.

Old people who are better off financially usually go to private homes rather than local authority welfare homes. Such homes vary widely in size, facilities provided, and cost. At one extreme some are extremely expensive; at the other extreme some are very bad and fairly cheap. A frequent regrettable feature is the absence of night staff.

A kind of asylum of which we have recently heard much is the hospice. This word used to be applied to a house of rest for pilgrims or travellers, often under the auspices of a religious order, or sometimes to a home for the destitute. A hospice is now usually a home for the dying and there has been much talk of the 'hospice movement' both in Britain and the United States. We have all read accounts of hospices where, because of the atmosphere of hope, the kindness of the staff and the skilful use of drugs, people dying of cancer have achieved a pain-free state of tranquillity. It has been said that to spend one's last days in such a place is far better than in an acute hospital, where the staff naturally concentrate their attention on the patients who are likely to recover.

Hostels have been set up for the mentally disturbed, where they can live a protected life and have someone to call on for help yet go out to work. In principle, this is immeasurably better than keeping people in a mental hospital (or prison) indefinitely. The degree of success achieved clearly depends to a large extent on the quality of the staff who run the hostels. In can be hoped that social misfits and perhaps recidivists will be enabled to live not too intolerable lives and to give something to society.

THE PROPER USE OF RESOURCES

Although the phrase 'infinite demand: finite resources' has been so often and so wrongly applied to the curing side of the health service, it can rightly be applied to the caring side. There is hardly a ceiling to the money which could properly be spent. If extreme poverty could be abolished that alone would improve the situation enormously. For the aged poor tend to live in the worst accommodation, number of old people, tend to live in the worst accommodation, often lacking heating and indoor sanitation. Improving this accommodation would help to keep them out of an asylum.

Few like the idea of an asylum, for its very existence seems to imply failure. And few doctors want to be associated with an asylum. Before and after the war psycho-analysts and others who did what was called psychotherapy were heard to make disdainful comments about those inferior medical people who merely did 'custodial' duties in the loony bins. The phrase 'once a lunatic; always a lunatic' was said to embody the attitude of the old-fashioned medical superintendent of the mental hospital. The more junior doctors in the mental hospital world resented the suggestion that they just did nothing except interview relatives and deal with organic diseases which the inmates of the mental hospital developed. They naturally wanted to be active and to treat mental disease in its 'early' stages before patients became lifelong inmates of the hospital. Likewise there was a great surge of activity in the geriatric field.

But, as I have endeavoured to show, there remains a vast need for asylums - a need which gets greater as the average age of the population rises. Many old people, living alone in squalor and neglect, and other old people sharing small houses with resentful relatives would be far better off in an asylum.

The staff of an asylum, whether it be a longterm mental hospital ward, a geriatric ward, a welfare home, a hospice, or a hostel, need a minimum of medical technology and a maximum of loving care. Few doctors should have to feel resentful that they are working in an asylum, because doctors are hardly wanted there. Other kinds of highly skilled staff are not wanted either. Common sense and kindliness are the qualities mainly required.

When Secretaries of State for the Social Services have suggested that resources should be diverted to the severely mentally defective or other unfortunates who need care, there has often been loud resentment in medical circles. Among the doctors the pressure is nearly all to spend more and more on the curing side, especially for advanced technology. If only we doctors would realize that we can benefit only a few people in certain specified circumstances, recent trends could be reversed and it would become possible to increase very greatly the resources devoted to the all-important caring.

SUMMARY

(1) Most care is in practice provided by relatives and neighbours. Financial inducements could encourage relatives to continue to look after the old, rather than move them to an asylum.
(2) There remains a great and increasing need for asylums, especially for the mentally disturbed and the senile geriatric. The belief, common in the recent past, that by energetic action by psychiatrists and geriatricians the need for asylum could be largely abolished is absurd..And the DHSS policy of phasing out the old longterm mental hospitals was mistaken.
(3) Most asylums need not be in hospitals. Rather should there be welfare homes (with an admission standard lower than at present), hospices, and special hostels.
(4) The phrase 'infinite demand: finite resources' is truly applicable to the caring side of the Health Service. Vastly more resources should be devoted to it.

References

1. Falck, H.S. and Kane, M.K. (1971). *It can't be Home. (Maryland: Department of Health, Education, and Welfare, Public Health Service, Health Services and Mental Health Administration, National Institute of Mental Health).*
2. Williams, D. (1979). *Br. Med. J.* **1,** 264
3. Bailey, K.C. (1979). *Br. Med. J.* **1,** 264

7

The Delivery of Medical Care

In Chapter 4 I observed that the phrase 'Prevention is better than cure' is a truism. I also commented that in the affluent societies much illness is related to indulgence, in food, tobacco, alcohol and lack of exercise. If people would avoid smoking altogether, restrain their food intake so that they were always slim, drink alcohol in moderation and not drink before driving, and take regular vigorous exercise their state of health would be vastly improved. In addition, accidents must largely be prevented by self-discipline - and accidents are the commonest cause of death and permanent disability in the young. In all this, the individual doctor dealing with his individual patients has almost no part to play. His one useful preventative role is by encouraging vaccination. There is a commonly held belief, especially in the United States, that regular physical examination with various investigations will improve health. In practice, this is liable to do far more harm than good.

The traditional function of the doctor has been to attend to people when they develop symptoms. This is still the main function of the clinician, though other kinds of doctor have other functions.

Before anaesthetics made surgery practicable, doctors were impotent to influence the course of virtually every malady; all they could do was to relieve symptoms with opiates and reassure and console. In practice, they gave all kinds of 'treatment' - bleeding, resting, purging, blistering, starving and a variety of hideous mixtures — which worsened the prospects of recovery. Even when surgery had become established, it was only relevant to a tiny proportion of episodes of illness. After the therapeutic revolution, doctors could do much more, but even today most maladies are influenced little or not at all by treatment. This does not of course mean that doctors are useless in most circumstances. They can allay anxiety and explain to patients the nature of their condition and sometimes give symptomatic relief. Nevertheless, only in those uncommon situations when treatment influences the course of illness is it important that the patient should consult a doctor. How can we best achieve this?

Even in the most sophisticated and highly educated societies it is impossible to lay down guidelines to the public which tell them when a doctor should be consulted. In practice, the only means of dealing with the problem is to enable everyone who feels unwell to see a doctor (though it may still be reasonable to put out propaganda to the public pointing out that, say, there is usually no point in seeing a doctor for a common cold). In the affluent societies doctors are as a rule available, though it may be difficult to get in touch with one.

Another important practical question is: What kinds of doctors should be directly available? In the United States and many European countries the people can go directly to a specialist whereas in Britain they can as a rule only see a general practitioner, though in a few circumstances, such as the suspicion of venereal disease, there is direct access to a specialist. Which is the best arrangement for first contact care?

Because of the increasing complexity and rapid advances in medicine it has been said that no-one can master more than a small fraction of it. The very concept of the general practitioner, who tries to know a little about everything, is, therefore, absurd. But if there are no general practitioners, how can the patient know which specialist he should approach? If he has a pain in his chest he cannot know whether he should see a heart or a lung or a rheumatic specialist - or a psychiatrist. And many patients have multiple symptoms. This is one important reason for the continued existence of general practitioners.

But the over-riding reason in favour of the general practitioner is that many maladies, especially long-standing ones, provide a general, not a specialist problem. A common symptom is a general malaise, masquerading as being 'run-down' or 'not myself' or 'always tired'. If this is of recent origin it may be due to some organic disease, but when long-standing it suggests an emotional basis, with depression predominant. Numerous patients complain of 'rheumatism', which may mean many different symptoms but frequently means indefinite widespread aches and pains - rheumatism 'everywhere'. Perhaps the commonest of all symptoms is headache. In very few patients is this due to any disease of the head structures (unless migraine is said to be such a disease). Especially when long-standing and continuous, headache usually reflects the state of the psyche; when of short duration it may reflect various disturbances, including fever, exposure to the sun, a loaded rectum, an alcoholic carouse, or some acute psychological trauma. Children commonly present with fever for no apparent cause (and frequently they recover without any better diagnosis than that of a 'flu-like illness').

Even when dealing with a patient's problem which the expertise of the specialist can help to elucidate, the doctor who has a generalist approach may still be best. A common problem is the middle-aged man with pain in the chest which may be related to myocardial ischaemia. The cardiologist who sees such a patient may concentrate his attention on the e.c.g. findings and other investigations, perhaps including coronary angiography, and ignore the patient. Indeed, William Evans[1] (1959) a famous cardiologist, urged that, when dealing with patients who may have cardiac pain 'less reliance must be placed on the patient's description of his illness and greater reliance on the electrocardiogram, which should be the final arbiter'. This approach inevitably leads to two errors: concluding that pain cannot be cardiac because the e.c.g. is normal (and no doubt this often does no harm) and concluding that pain must be cardiac because the e.c.g. is abnormal (and this can have disastrous effects). For just as many people have e.c.g. abnormalities who are symptom-free, so others have these abnormalities accompanying non-cardiac pain. Moreover, a patient who has had a cardiac infarct is likely in consequence to have suffered severe psychological trauma and later may have left mammary aching and other psychosomatic symptoms. The cardiologist who makes the e.c.g. 'the final arbiter' will wrongly conclude that this pain is due to myocardial ischaemia, whereas the generalist who looks at the whole patient will reach the correct conclusion and give appropriate reassurance. The general practitioner should be the generalist *in excelsis,* though not all GPs succeed in this respect. Some of them too ignore the patient and concentrate on the presenting symptom or the bit of the body from whence it arises.

A corollary of this is that all clinicians should be generalists much of the time. When the abdominal surgeon is performing a highly selective vagotomy his specialized knowledge and experience enable him to do this properly. But when he is talking to a patient with a suspected duodenal ulcer in the out-patient department, and considering whether or not to advise highly selective vagotomy, he should not just concentrate on the patient's description of his pain and the X-ray and endoscopic appearances. He should also sit back and look at the whole man against his background. How much disastrous surgery has been performed by surgeons who have failed to do this!

There are also great practical advantages for the ordinary citizen in having someone who is 'my doctor'. When he is taken ill he does not have to wonder or discuss with his family and friends where he should turn for help; he knows that he has his own doctor, in whom he usually has trust (though if he wants advice urgently he may have to see the duty doctor in the first instance). No doubt this trust is mainly dependent on neighbourhood gossip or on the fact that he finds the doctor is a likeable man who inspires confidence, but it nevertheless means much to the patient that he feels this trust.

The advantages of general practice can be combined with a degree of specialization by having different doctors for different age groups. Indeed, in the Court Report and elsewhere GP paediatricians have been advocated. There has been no suggestion yet that there should be GP geriatricians. The GP paediatrician can acquire a special knowledge of childhood maladies but he still remains a generalist who looks at the whole patient, and the patient (or his mother) does not have to decide which organ is responsible for the symptoms. On the other hand, this kind of specialization implies that parents and children have different GPs, which has obvious disadvantages.

The British system in which the doctor of first contact is a general practitioner is, then, by far the best. And whatever technological advances are made in the future, this will remain true, since most maladies will always present a general, not a specialist, problem. In some parts of the world where the general practitioner has all but disappeared there have been many voices to regret his demise. This has happened in the United States. In 1969 the American Board of General Practice was created by the American Academy of General Practice and the Section on General Practice of the American Medical Association as a means to reversing the then current trends. But we understand that this effort has so far resulted in only qualified success.

THE NEED FOR SPECIALIZATION

The most obvious need for specialization among clinicians is provided by surgery. No-one should do difficult surgical operations on an occasional basis. And no surgeon can master the technique of all operations. As the field of surgery has widened increasing specialization within surgery has become justified. As to just how far this should go is debatable. The ultimate degree of specialization is that every surgeon only performs one particular operation. This would be absurd.

The disadvantages of extreme surgical specialization are firstly, that the surgeon finds his work so monotonous that he skimps his operations, secondly, that it is often impossible to know which operation is indicated until the patient has been opened and thirdly, that working in a narrow field tends to warp the surgeon's judgment. Even with a 'reasonable' degree of specialization it becomes difficult for a surgeon to retain a balanced attitude. When a surgeon is doing an operation he is using his particular expertise, but when he is considering whether or not to advise an operation he should be both specialist and generalist. And as a rule the longer the symptoms have been present, the more should his decision rest on his general study of the whole patient.

Radiotherapy is unique because it is a specialty of treatment. A patient referred to a surgeon is not automatically advised operation, but when a patient with advanced malignant disease is referred to a radiotherapist, how often does he advise that neither radiotherapy nor cancer chemotherapy should be given? I do not recall a single such instance among patients referred by me. Many radiotherapists defend the giving of treatment nearly always on the ground that the patient has had his hopes raised by the prospect of the healing rays and that to dash these hopes would be cruel. The surgeon who performed a useless operation because he did not wish to dash the patient's hopes would be condemned. Why should the opposite argument be valid for radiotherapists? It cannot be argued that operation is necessarily a serious procedure whereas radiotherapy or chemotherapy are trivial. On the contrary, a quick 'open and shut' laparotomy is often trivial whereas the side-effects of radiotherapy and chemotherapy can be most unpleasant.

For only a few conditions, including chorionepithelioma, Hodgkin's disease and acute lymphatic leukaemia, are radiotherapy or chemotherapy actually curative, and many victims even of these conditions in the end die of them. Otherwise, these remedies are palliative. They may still give a worthwhile remission, notably for some of the reticuloses, some testicular tumours, and neuroblastoma. But many patients treated by radiotherapists have such conditions as inoperable carcinoma of bronchus, cerebral glioma, or multiple metastases. The treatment of these patients is sometimes justified by anecdotes of similar cases who made spectacular improvement. If there were a significant number of such cases and firm evidence that the improvement was due to treatment, we could justify giving most patients the benefit of the doubt. But the proportion of patients who do well is very small. Most are given unpleasant side-effects followed by a deterioration in the quality of life and often with no prolongation of life.

Far more radiotherapy and chemotherapy are given than should be given. An important reason for this is that radiotherapy is a specialty of treatment. These remedies should be given only to those patients for whom there is a reasonable hope either of cure or of prolonged and striking improvement. This is only likely to be achieved, it is to be feared, because physicians and surgeons decline to refer cases to radiotherapy departments. Until radiotherapists refuse to treat a substantial proportion of patients referred to them they can hardly be considered to be consultants. Rather are they technical advisers with expert knowledge about malignant disease and the effects of various rays and toxic drugs who leave it to others to decide whether the treatment should be given.

The non-clinical specialities of radiology, anaesthetics and the various branches of pathology can all be justified. With the increasing elaboration of the equipment used in these fields, no-one can properly master them as a part-time occupation. A question which these specialties pose is whether all those who work in these fields need be qualified doctors. In many countries most anaesthetists are not medical graduates and in Britain an increasing proportion of chemical pathologists are science graduates. There are evident advantages in all these specialists having a knowledge of medicine, and this is especially so if they are radiologists or haematologists. But if few were medical graduates the situation would not necessarily be worse than it is now.

PHYSICIANS

The main justification for the specialties so far considered is the need to master difficult and constantly changing techniques. Most physicians do not need to master any difficult techniques. The main exception to this rule are the gastro-enterologists, who become expert at endoscopy. But the chief clinical reason (though there may also be reasons of research) for endoscopy is to determine whether or not surgery is indicated. If there is no question of surgery there is little justification in putting the patient to the discomfort of endoscopy. Much the same considerations apply to cardiac catheterization and coronary arteriography. The reason why cardiologists do them is because surgery may be recommended. The main techniques acquired by nephrologists or hepatologists are the means to obtain biopsy specimens. But this is easily learnt. And the important part of the process, examining the specimen under a microscope, is carried out by the pathologist. Most chest physicians do not perform bronchoscopies; instead they pass the patients on to surgeons. If a physician does a bronchoscopy himself this should also be because of the possibility of an operation.

Patients are referred to the out-patient department to see a physician because the GP wishes for help either in diagnosis or management or because the patient or his relatives demand a second opinion. It has been said that patients have a 'right' to see a specialist if they so wish. Many GPs act as if they had this right, as they always give way to the demand for a second opinion. This is an abnegation of responsibility by the GP. If he believes there is no point in someone seeing a consultant he should say so and as a rule the patient will accept this. A few patients, or their relatives, will not of course agree that referral is unnecessary and if they are very persistent and difficult the GP can hardly be blamed for yielding. The only right the patient has if he does not accept his GP's advice is to change his GP.

Perhaps the average consultant physician derives his greatest satisfaction in the out-patient department by making a precise diagnosis in an obscure case. In my student days stories used to be told of the giants of the previous generation who had done this in cases who had baffled all the lesser lights in the hospital. But in truth this kind of diagnostic tour de force only happens infrequently; most patients who are obscure to one doctor remain obscure to others. And the occasions when this diagnosis benefits the patient are rare indeed. I analysed the last 450 out-patients I saw before retiring[2] (Todd, 1978) and in only one who was referred to me because he was obscurely ill did the making of a diagnosis result in useful treatment. This was a man with osseous metastases from a carcinoma prostate. And this diagnosis was simply reached; the bone X-rays were characteristic and the acid phosphatase level was enormous. The patient responded in a most dramatic manner to stilboestrol. Most medical patients who are much benefited by the making of a precise diagnosis are the acutely ill admitted as emergencies.

In any case, as I pointed out in Chapter 2 (p. 24) the idea that if one is clever enough and learned enough all patients can be fitted into a neat pigeon hole called an entity is false. Entities are devised by men; nature is more complex. Moreover, diagnosis does not just consist of attaching a label to a patient, especially when there is a long history and multiple symptoms. A patient's malaise is not just determined by the state of a bodily organ; it is also determined by his psyche, and that in turn is related to his temperament and his circumstances. The chronically complaining patient should be diagnosed not by a word but by a sentence, such as, 'Habitually worrying man with a boring job and a nagging wife who has myocardial ischaemia not interfering with his ordinary activities, but about which he is very worried'.

Most patients who are referred to consultants for help with treatment have surgical conditions. For medical treatment is as a rule straightforward. Among the patients who are referred to physicians for therapeutic reasons are diabetics, the obese and hypertensives. Could not GPs manage such patients themselves? Many GPs in fact do so.

The commonest diabetic is the maturity onset overweight type. We all know what is the correct treatment - the patient should make a large reduction in his calorie intake for the rest of his life. The practical problem presented by such a patient is that he fails to restrict his diet (though - astonishingly - books on diabetes hardly ever mention this problem, much less solve it). The least unsuccessful way of dealing with this situation is for the patient to join a self-help club, such as the Weight Watchers. Otherwise, the GP can probably do just as well as can the consultant, even with the aid of a hospital dietitian. The same considerations apply to the obese who are not diabetics and most of them remain obese, whatever course is adopted, though many achieve considerable temporary weight reductions.

Most GPs refer newly diagnosed juvenile onset diabetics because the treatment is thought complex and it is widely taken for granted that such patients should all be admitted to hospital for 'initial stabilization'. I have long maintained[3] that this is wholly mistaken (Todd, 1972). The very phrase 'initial stabilization' is absurd because most diabetics when first started on insulin are not stable. They are best controlled while living their usual lives. The main function of the doctor is to teach these people how to look after themselves by adjusting their insulin dose and by eating and exercising appropriately. As to how steady they should be advised to maintain their carbohydrate intake is debatable and whatever advice is given, few follow it exactly. In any case, if the amount of exercise taken is varied, so should be the carbohydrate intake. In so far as diabetic complications are minimized by maintaining the blood sugar as near normal as possible the best practical means of achieving this is probably to put the patient on two doses of insulin daily and tell him to take the biggest dose which does not cause unacceptable hypoglycaemia.

Although there are no doubt grounds why GPs should refer juvenile onset diabetics to hospital, the GP who is willing to take the time and trouble can manage the situation himself. And there seems little point in diabetics on insulin attending a diabetic clinic every 3 or 6 months when, according to the testimony of many, they see a different doctor on each occasion and have a random blood sugar estimated. Many of the most successful diabetics I have known have seen neither a GP nor a consultant for years. They have learnt to look after themselves and have merely left requests for a prescription at intervals with the GP's receptionist.

Some GPs regularly refer hypertensive patients whilst others do not. Here, either diagnosis or treatment may be thought to be grounds for obtaining a consultant's opinion. The chances of discovering a possibly remediable condition, such as phaeo-chromocytoma or renal artery stenosis, are so minute that the sophisticated investigations needed to diagnose these conditions are probably not justified except in the young, if even then. Otherwise, the important decision is whether to give treatment and if so which treatment. The GP should be able to answer these questions nearly as well as can the consultant.

It may be thought that the consultant physician should set an example to his GP colleagues by giving the very best treatment. No doubt the consultant will be less likely to prescribe anorectics or thyroxin for the obese, sulphonylurea compounds for the obese diabetic, and methyldopa for the octogenarian hypertensive than will the GP. But the difficulty here is to discover objective criteria to determine which is the best treatment. It is well to remember some of the treatment recommended by the most eminent physicians only 2 or 3 decades ago. Then, the luckless victims of cardiac infarction were kept at absolute rest for a few days, in bed for 6 or more weeks and encouraged to live semi-invalid lives thereafter. And those with duodenal ulcer (most of whom without treatment would soon have a remission, perhaps for months or years) would be put to bed on a diet of citrated milk and every week additions to the diet such as finely minced steamed fish, rusks to be well chewed, sieved apples, and bread and butter pudding, until after 6 weeks a life-long diet which lacked spices, skins, and anything roast or fried would be advised. Similar examples could be multiplied indefinitely.

Apart from making an occasional important diagnosis and giving suggestions about treatment, I used to feel that my most valuable function with out-patients was to reassure. In at least one third of cases the psyche appeared to be largely or wholly responsible for the symptoms, and in many of the others it played a large part. As to how much benefit can be given in this way it is impossible to say; there are no controlled trials in this field. Nevertheless, when a patient has recently developed somatic anxiety symptoms (such as left mammary aching, palpitation, unsteadiness, and difficulty in filling the lungs) which he fears are due to heart disease, a categorical promise that his heart is fine and that such symptoms are due to anxiety often gives him immediate relief and his symptoms may well disappear and not return. Perhaps a substantial proportion of patients with somatic anxiety symptoms can be given some help in this way. Of course, this kind of reassurance can just as well be given by the GP though some patients may more readily, if quite unjustifiably, accept reassurance from a consultant than a GP.

One of the accepted activities of the consultant physician is research. However, the most important medical research is that which may result in the cure or prevention of disease. Nearly all such research is carried out by backroom scientists. Clinicians become concerned only when the backroom scientists produce a new drug or a new apparatus to be tried on man.

Research that clinicians can do is to observe and study groups of patients. Over the years much has been learnt by this kind of study. GPs can also do such research. The GP who does a 30-year follow-up of his patients with rheumatoid arthritis, peptic ulcer and other variable maladies can much improve our understanding of them, whereas hospital consultants tend only to deal with those worst affected by these conditions, so their observations are often biased. It used to be said that multiple sclerosis is in the end always fatal. The evident reason for this depressing conclusion was that the minor cases with life-long remissions were not seen by the eminent neurologists who wrote the textbooks.

GENERAL PHYSICIAN OR SPECIALIST?

There has been an endless debate for years as to whether or not consultant physicians should cover the whole field of medicine or confine their attention to some system. It has often been said that the increasing complexity of medicine has made the old-time general physician obsolete. But, leaving aside neurologists, dermatologists, and some chest physicians and rheumatologists, physicians in Britain are still mostly appointed as general physicians, though often with a 'special interest'. Their in-patients admitted as emergencies (and nearly all those in acute medical wards should be emergencies) are put under each physician on specified days, so they all have the usual mix of patients with pain in the chest, overdoses, strokes, respiratory infection etc. Indeed, most of such patients are not helped by the expertise of the consultant and do not need (though they often have) sophisticated investigations. The essential reason for their being in hospital is that they are acutely ill and cannot be looked after at home.

I concluded above that most patients most of the time are best looked after by a GP because they present a general problem. The patients for whom the GP wants a second opinion may also present a general problem. Some are generally unwell with multiple symptoms; others are psychologically disturbed with somatic symptoms. The general physician is likely to handle such patients better than the physician who considers himself to be a nephrologist or a gastro-enterologist. Indeed, the physician who says, as some do, that he is only interested in hearts or endocrine organs or some other system is likely to be a disaster. Even if a physician is a cardiologist or an endocrinologist he is, or should be, acting as a general physician most of the time and should look at patients as people. For the vast majority of people referred to the out-patient department all the advanced technology of the specialist physician - endoscopy, coronary arteriography, renal biopsy and the rest — has no place (though it is often wrongly used).

Among the worst of the errors made by doctors (see Chapter 8, p.137) has been the wrong attribution of symptoms to disease, actual or hypothetical, of the system from which the symptoms are arising. Belly symptoms were attributed to visceroptosis, chronic appendicitis, chronic gastritis or, more recently, hiatus hernia. Backache was attributed to retroverted uterus and headache to errors of refraction, sinusitis, cervical spondylopathy, or hypertension. The specialists who concentrate their whole attention on their own region are most likely to make such errors.

There is no doubt a place for the physician who makes a special study of a particular system, provided he retains his general outlook. This may be so in research institutes, in renal units where patients are having dialysis or transplants, and in cardiological units where patients are assessed with a view to surgery. But the value of a physician is derived far more from his general qualities than from his special knowledge. Such qualities as good judgement, the ability to see the patient as a whole, the ability to see all aspects of a problem in the right perspective and the ability to weigh up evidence are far more important than detailed knowledge of some rare syndrome.

In spite of all this we often hear that many more specialist physicians are needed. Not every patient with migraine or epilepsy is seen by a neurologist, so more neurologists should be appointed. The rheumatic complaints, and especially backache, are responsible for much absence from work, yet rheumatologists are very thin on the ground and (it is habitually said in the lay press) doctors are no use in dealing with backache. But the very idea that patients are necessarily better off by seeing some hyper-specialist is absurd. What we need is a cure for rheumatoid arthritis, not the multiplication of rheumatologists. We also need a cure, or a means of prevention, for all kinds of backache, though it is hardly conceivable that this will ever be achieved.

The main need for clinical specialization is, then, for surgeons and radiotherapists, because their work involves difficult techniques. We also need consultant physicians, some of whom are specialists though all should retain a general approach. But if we had enough competent general practitioners with suitable back-up services, and if the public could be convinced that a specialist is not necessarily best, we could manage with fewer consultant physicians than we have now.

Similar considerations apply to psychiatrists and geriatricians. Psychiatrists do not have to master any techniques. Patients are referred to them for advice about management and treatment. The one kind of treatment which demands much expertise is psychotherapy.

Many of the intelligentsia take it for granted that psychotherapy, and in particular psycho-analysis, is beneficial. It is indeed remarkable how psycho-analytic concepts have been accepted by some of the most articulate and educated sections of the community, especially in the United States. This is considered in Chapter 9, p. 191.

Without doubt, simple psychotherapy in the form of reassurance can give immediate relief to people with certain kinds of anxiety. If a man has recently developed unpleasant head sensations which he fears are due to a cerebral tumour, the categorical promise that he cannot possibly have a cerebral tumour will probably rid him of his worry and his symptoms. Admittedly, if he is not reassured, he will in time cease to worry and lose his symptoms anyway. On the other hand, if a patient has a long-standing conviction that he has some dread disease, in particular venereal disease, this kind of reassurance is usually a waste of time.

In practice, this simple kind of effective psychotherapy is given by GPs and physicians rather than by psychiatrists. The patients referred to them have a disturbance much more profound than a recent worry about health. The main treatment given by most psychiatrists is a psychotropic drug. There has been a continuous debate as to the benefit given by these drugs. Although there are good grounds for concluding that psychotropic drugs sometimes give worthwhile help, they are often apparently ineffective or still leave the patient desperately unhappy and worried. These same drugs are also prescribed on a huge scale, probably a grossly excessive scale, by GPs. Although the psychiatrist has much more experience in their use than have GPs, it seems most doubtful whether this experience helps the psychiatrist to prescribe 'better'; in this field there are too many variables to make it possible to lay down a best scheme of treatment. And, in any case, psychiatrists give conflicting advice.

Although psychiatrists no doubt give helpful advice to GPs the benefit they can give is, like that usually given by physicians, quite modest. We constantly hear of the shortage of psychiatrists and of the enormous waiting lists for out-patient appointments. This does not justify any increase in the number of psychiatrists; it implies that GPs should be much more restrained in referring patients to psychiatrists.

Before the Second World War there were no geriatricians in Britain; now most hospitals have them. But very few young doctors look forward to a career in geriatrics. Many geriatricians hoped to become consultant physicians, failed to do so and decided to become geriatricians, and nearly two-thirds of senior registrars are from overseas.

One underlying reason for the expansion in geriatrics was that 'the old' were thought to be getting a raw deal from society. They were poor, neglected, and forgotten. Indeed, old people living on nothing beyond their old-age pension and supplementary benefits were and still are the very poorest of the population. It was also commonly stated that old people were badly treated when ill. They would be tucked up in bed, either by their relatives or in hospital, because they were conveniently out of the way and in consequence they would develop bed-sores, contractures, and apathy, which was only relieved when they died. Of course until recently it was a fundamental medical belief that people who had almost any illness - fever, childbirth, peptic ulcer, rheumatoid arthritis, coronary thrombosis, and operation - should be kept in bed for weeks. With luck, this caused transient harm to the young and middle-aged; only the old were killed by it. But this belief in the universal value of bed-rest is dead. One now hears stories of old people who are constantly bullied into activity when their only wish is to be left alone.

No doubt a great deal more resources should be devoted to all the underprivileged members of society, including the old. The old should have more money and, when they become infirm, more help to keep their independence while still living in their own homes, which nearly all wish to do. There should also be a great increase in asylum accommodation (see Chapter 6)

But all this has little to do with geriatrics. Of course, old people should constantly be encouraged by everyone involved - doctors, physiotherapists, nurses, health visitors, relatives and friends - to keep active, but the supreme driving force always has been and always will be the personality of the old person. Geriatricians admit that little can be done for those with senile dementia (and we now have unfortunate psycho-geriatricians to deal with them). In practice, the senile dements provide the intractable problem; there is little difficulty in making satisfactory arrangements for old people with normal intellects, even when they have severe physical incapacity.

Geriatricians may claim that only by working among the old can the necessary expertise to treat them properly be acquired. As people become older, it is said, diseases subtly change in their presentation and old people characteristically have multiple pathology. It follows, therefore, that physicians untrained in geriatric medicine are liable to make diagnostic errors and especially to make one diagnosis instead of two or three. But a general physician would have to be singularly blind and stupid to make such elementary errors. The middle-aged or even the young may have multiple chronic pathology - hallux valgus, knock knee, obesity, varicose veins, ingrowing toenail etc., along with something more sinister. We should merely be wary of diagnosing two independent acute conditions simultaneously. And this wariness should be applied just as much to the old as to the young.

In any case, most patients, especially women, admitted as emergencies into acute medical wards under general physicians are of geriatric age. And this is also true of many of those referred to out-patients. In most hospitals the wards under the geriatrician's care are largely occupied by longterm patients, most of whom remain there until they die. This is no doubt a contributory explanation for the unpopularity of geriatrics as a specialty. Geriatricians themselves naturally tend to take the view that many, if not all, acutely sick people of geriatric age should be admitted under them. But if this became the standard practice, there would be a revolt by the general physicians. There have been suggestions of a compromise - that physicians and geriatricians should admit alternate acutely sick people of geriatric age under their care. But if this became the normal pattern, the obvious question would follow: 'Why not abolish the distinction between geriatricians and physicians and once more appoint just physicians?'

It has been said that if general physicians were put in charge of longterm geriatric wards they would mostly do no more than visit them occasionally and rush round the patients at high speed (as many did in the former local authority hospitals). This criticism implies that those in longterm geriatric wards need a great deal of medical attention. But if they have been admitted there for the right reasons - that is, they need an asylum because they cannot be looked after in their own homes and are too infirm for local authority homes - it is absurd to say that they should have the kind of intense medical attention given to the occupants of acute awards. An excellent way of dealing with their medical requirements would be to appoint general practitioners on a sessional basis (as is already done to some extent).

There are, then, good grounds for abolishing the specialty of geriatrics altogether. The only medical care needed by most old people most of the time is the same as that needed by the rest of the community - the attention of a general practitioner. When they have some condition remediable by surgery, they need the same surgeons as does everyone else (and no-one has suggested that we should have geriatric surgeons). And on those rare occasions when they have an acute medical condition for which sophisticated investigations (with the possibility of spectacular treatment) are appropriate, they need just the same physicians as does everyone else.

PAYING FOR MEDICAL CARE

The traditional way of paying the doctor is by fee for item of service. In Britain before the NHS this was the way by which most doctors were paid, except by panel patients. Some old doctors look back with nostalgic longing to those halcyon days. Then, the kindly old GP would 'forget' to charge his very poor patients, who would perhaps pay him with a gift of vegetables. Consultants tended to vary the size of their fee according to the degree of affluence of the patient (though many attacked this practice) and they would not charge clergymen at all. By earning money from the rich in this way they gave their time 'free' to serve the poor who attended the hospital. This Robin Hood principle was always popular.

In spite of the fact that we have now had the NHS for over 30 years, many doctors still believe that fee for item of service is the normal and natural way, as well as being the fairest way, of paying the doctor. Under that system the doctor is paid for the work he actually does, whereas with any other system some doctors work twice as hard, or half as hard, as do others for the same money. There has always been a large element in the British Medical Association which has pressed for fee for item of service. An especially beneficial effect of this system would be, it is said, to encourage GPs to do more for their patients. They would sew up cuts, syringe ears, and inject varicose veins, rather than, as so many are alleged to do, offload as much as possible onto the hospital service.

The supreme objection to fee for item of service is that it encourages unnecessary investigation, treatment, and visits. The surgeon who is paid £100 if he takes out tonsils and nothing if he does· not do so will be apt to find reasons for advising tonsillectomy. If a physician is paid extra for doing an electrocardiogram, he will hardly be human if he does not do so, for this cannot do the patient any harm and, in any case, there is a common belief that electrocardiograms should be done as routine. And the GP who is paid extra if he gives a prescription may salve his conscience by prescribing something harmless and saying to himself that the patient will be pleased and gain from the placebo effect.

In Britain there could be no conceivable possibility of persuading the Government to have a fee for item of service system without a ceiling on total expenditure. This would involve an army of bureaucrats to run the system and the dishonest doctors who did too much would gain at the expense of the honest ones.

The protagonists of fee for item of service sometimes say that to insinuate that doctors would do needless operations and give other wrong treatment is an insult to that great majority of honest doctors. No doubt few if any surgeons would excise an eye or amputate a leg just to make money. And few physicians or GPs would give a course of gold or penicillamine without good grounds. But the indications for many investigations and much treatment are most indefinite. There are probably no compelling grounds for tonsillectomy. The arguments for operation on varicose veins are questionable. Women who are approaching the menopause are often anxious to have a hysterectomy; whether or not the surgeon should give way to this pressure is arguable. The indications for one of the latest operations, coronary bypass surgery, are most uncertain. Vast numbers of investigations are often done as routine. And among drugs only iron, cyanacobalamin, insulin, thyroxine and a few others have clear-cut indications. To claim that in this uncertain territory financial considerations would not greatly influence decisions is ridiculous.

Those who favour the fee for item of service system sometimes say that other systems might be satisfactory if we were all wholly virtuous. But human nature being what it is, financial inducements are needed to encourage even doctors to give of their best. Knowing that if they work harder they will make more money they will indeed work harder. Human nature, therefore, is so depraved that financial inducements are continually needed, yet at the same time the medical profession has such high ideals that doctors will not do unnecessary operations or give unnecessary treatment for money. In any case, the very idea that doctors should be encouraged to be active is misguided. Our great fault has always been that we have not left well alone, but have given all sorts of misguided treatment, often with lethal effects.

My conclusion from all this is that fee for item of service is the worst possible system of payment. When no-one else is involved except the patient there is at least some inducement not to do too much - the patient's unwillingness to pay. But when the money is provided by the state, or equally by an insurance firm, this slight safeguard disappears. There may still be a few special circumstances when fee for item of service is not wholly objectionable. Anaesthetists, for example, might be paid in this way, since they do not decide whether or not the operation should be done. And fees for vaccination are legitimate.

Originally all the doctors in the NHS hospital service were paid a salary, either for working wholetime or on a sessional basis. To me this was the best and most civilized system of payment. Then in 1970 overtime payments for junior staff were introduced. At present strenuous efforts are being made by doctor's representatives to bring in various extra duty payments for consultants. All such payments put a premium upon dishonesty. Even those doctors who are normally highly scrupulous would hardly be human if, when they saw their colleagues making extra money in devious ways, they did not follow suit. One can only hope, if without conviction, that in the end we will all again be paid a salary for doing a job.

GPs in the NHS have always been mainly paid according to the number of patients on their lists. And there is no immediate prospect of any change in this system. Although there would be some advantages if GPs were paid by salary, the present system at least provides no incentives for making extra visits and giving unnecessary injections and prescriptions. Indeed, as was noted above, it may well encourage idle GPs to offload onto casualty departments simple problems which they could easily deal with themselves.

SUMMARY

(1) The doctor of first contact should be a general practitioner. He can deal with most medical problems, many of which are of a general nature.
(2) Specialization among clinicians is needed to master difficult techniques. This is mainly relevant to surgery and radiotherapy.
(3) Physicians have to master few techniques. Whether or not they have a special interest, they should all be generalists most of the time.
(4) Psychiatrists can only give modest help and we need no increase in their number.
(5) There is no convincing need for a separate specialty of geriatrics.
(6) The worst method of paying the doctor is fee for item of service. Overtime and most other extra duty payments encourage dishonesty. Hospital doctors are best paid by salary.

References

1. Evans, W. (1959). *Br. Med. J.*, **1**, 249
2. Todd, J.W. (1978). *Br. Med. J.*, **1**, 417
3. Todd, J.W. (1972). *J. R. Coll. Physicians*, **7**, 77

8

The Errors of Medicine

Throughout this book I repeatedly refer to the errors of medicine - the absurd theories, the futile and damaging treatments, the excessive investigations, the failure to look at the patient as a person, and the rest. In the present chapter I shall look at these errors at a deeper level, in the hope of discovering why we have made so many of them.

ERRONEOUS THEORIES OF AETIOLOGY

Theories of aetiology are at two levels: firstly, hypothesizing the cause of symptoms and secondly, when there is some undoubted pathological process, hypothesizing the cause of the process.

At the first level errors are made because symptoms are wrongly attributed to a non-existent pathological process or to an incidental pathological process or physiological variation which happens to be present. In the recent past there were many imaginary pathological processes. Perhaps the most familiar was 'fibrositis'. A decade or two ago this was said to be the commonest cause of absence from work, according to the Ministry of Health statistics. The term was first employed by Sir William Gowers in 1904. He suggested that lumbago was a 'hyperplastic inflammation' of insufficient degree to produce the induration or suppuration which are the manifestations of cellulitis and he called this 'fibrositis'. Stockman (1920)[1] established the pathological basis of 'fibrositis' by photomicrographs of the 'fibrositic nodule'. He observed: 'It seems at least likely that these focal fibroses are due to small colonies of microbes invading the tissue and causing a reaction which comparatively rapidly destroys the invaders'. Although it is now widely accepted that 'fibrositis' does not exist, patients with pain which appears muscular are still often told by their doctors that they have 'fibrositis' and lay people often make this diagnosis themselves. And the term still appears in the most recent textbooks, perhaps between quotes to emphasize that the disease has no reality.

'Neuritis' used to be nearly as common a diagnosis as 'fibrositis'. Sometimes this term was applied to patients in whom there was an undoubted pathological process affecting the peripheral nerves, such as that accompanying diabetes or vitamin B_1 deficiency. The more appropriate term neuropathy is now usually employed here.

But many patients with pain, in the limbs especially, were said to have 'neuritis', or sometimes 'interstitial neuritis'. Those with sciatic pain which would now be diagnosed as 'prolapsed disc' were said to have 'sciatic neuritis'. And patients with arm pain which would now be thought to be due to cervical spondylopathy or the carpal tunnel syndrome were said to have 'brachial neuritis'. The pathological basis to this 'neuritis' was said to be an inflammation of the connective tissues which surround and bind together the nerve fibres into the nerve trunks.

One of the commonest causes of low backache used to be 'sacro-iliac strain'. This was a convenient kind of pathology to hypothesize, since even if a patient came to postmortem the sceptic could not prove that there had been no 'strain' of the sacro-iliac joints during life. 'Lumbo-sacral back strain' was another explanation of backache. Persistent ache in the right iliac fossa was attributed to 'chronic appendicitis'.

Pathological changes were regularly hypothesized to explain somatic symptoms which were, in truth, the manifestations of emotional disorder. Cardiac symptoms were attributed to 'myocarditis' or 'primary cardiac overstrain' (see p. 38). Even impotence was thought to be due to inflammation of the seminal vesicles. And dyspareunia was attributed to a congenitally tight vagina.

Among the abnormalities to which symptoms were wrongly attributed one of the most notorious was retroversion of the uterus, which in my student days was said to be the commonest cause of persistent low backache in women. Persistent or recurrent abdominal symptoms were attributed to ptosis of the abdominal contents - visceroptosis when it was believed that the entire gut was affected or gastroptosis or nephroptosis when the stomach or kidney alone were thought to be at fault. Abdominal symptoms were attributed to hyperchlorhydria (Reichmann's disease) or to hypochlorhydria or achlorhydria. Head sensations, such as giddiness, muzziness, or persistent dull ache, were thought to be caused by hypertension. Lassitude, insomnia, headache, and giddiness were said to be the symptoms of hypotension. Another common cause of headache was said to be astigmatism. Indeed, whereas minor astigmatism was believed to cause headache, gross astigmatism was said not to do so. One more familiar explanation of headache was sinusitis.

Theories of this kind may be thought to be merely of historic interest. Indeed, imaginative pathology, such as fibrositis, interstitial neuritis and sacro-iliac strain, is now almost dead, even though the diagnoses themselves linger on. But there still remains a tendency to attribute symptoms to some incidental abnormality.

A common diagnosis now made in dyspeptics is 'hiatus hernia'. When the cardiac sphincter is inadequate and a patient complains of retrosternal pain when lying down which is relieved on sitting up there are good grounds for diagnosing 'hiatus hernia' - or more accurately 'oesophagitis accompanying hiatus hernia'. But when a patient is being exhaustively investigated for dyspepsia and the radiologist keeps him in the head-down position for a long time, some reflux of barium is common. The symptoms are then all too easily attributed to 'hiatus hernia'. Even if the doctor does not make this error but the patient is told about the reflux, he himself may take it for granted that his troubles are due to an 'internal hernia'.

When women are found to have a haemoglobin level of, say, 10 g per 100 ml their various symptoms, such as lassitude, tiredness, and weakness may wrongly be attributed to 'anaemia'. Again, even if the doctor does not make this mistake but a patient is told that she has anaemia she will probably take it for granted that this explains her malaise. In fact, minor anaemia appears to be symptomless (though when the anaemia is due to some such sinister cause as carcinoma stomach there may be symptoms from this). In like manner, patients who are being correctly treated for pernicious anaemia may continue to 'suffer' from this condition and attribute incidental symptoms to it.

Headache and other head sensations are still often attributed to hypertension. Once more, even if the doctor does not say that this is so, if a patient knows that his blood pressure is raised he will probably assume that his head sensations are due to this. Indeed, if symptomless people are told they have high blood pressure they may soon cease to be symptomless. A corollary of this is that if a doctor discovers hypertension but considers that treatment is not indicated, he is justified in with holding the information from the patient that his blood pressure is raised. And if the doctor does inform the patient he should point out that headache, giddiness and other head sensations are not due to raised blood pressure. Headache is also still wrongly attributed to sinusitis.

THE CAUSE OF PATHOLOGICAL PROCESSES

The second great error in the field of aetiology is to make improper hypotheses as to the cause of pathological processes. Indeed, throughout history doctors have attempted to find some simple single explanation of a whole range of maladies. In the last century many conditions were attributed to 'strain', and as this state cannot be defined, no-one could prove that 'strain' was not responsible. 50 years ago, constipation with its associated 'intestinal auto-intoxication' was thought to be an important cause of diseases. In consequence, the public became obsessed with the state of its bowels and although doctors long ago ceased to believe in 'intestinal auto-intoxication' this obsession still persists. Sir William Arbuthnot Lane believed in this theory so fervently that he performed colectomies on numerous patients.

In my student days the great unifying hypothesis was toxic absorption from septic foci, though advanced thinkers were already beginning to deride it. Many of the maladies which we think are peculiarly obscure were explained in this way, including rheumatoid arthritis, ulcerative colitis, iritis, peptic ulcer, and multiple sclerosis. The same mechanism was hypothesized for 'fibrositis' and 'neuritis', so here there was a double error - imaginative pathology which was explained by hypothetical toxins. In consequence, many patients had various investigations to discover septic foci. One famous physician regularly admitted patients to 'search for sepsis'. If no septic focus was found, or if septic foci had been removed but the malady remained, the stools would be sent to the laboratory and a vaccine made from the cultures, which would be injected into the unfortunate patient in increasing doses.

Nearly 30 years ago the General Adaptation Syndrome swept through the world of medicine, largely as the result of Hans Selye's researches, and in a year or two disappeared almost without trace. According to the theory, various *stressors* (such as fright, pathogenic organisms, cold, muscular effort, trauma), as well as having specific actions on parts of the body, were also believed to have non-specific effects. As a result, the pituitary produces more corticotrophin and other hormones and the adrenal cortex in turn produces more corticosteroids. Some of the corticosteroids stimulate the proliferative ability and reactivity of connective tissues and others cause involution of connective tissue with a weakening of resistance to infection. Imperfections in this general adaptation process were thought to be a major cause of many maladies, notably much arterial disease and rheumatoid arthritis.

Another ambitious explanation of many bodily diseases is the psychosomatic theory. This is dealt with in Chapter 3, p.40. It is an ancient theory which had a surge of popularity after the Second World War, but is now declining.

Closely involved with the psychosomatic theory is the myth of the 'stress and strain of modern life'. A few years ago we repeatedly read, both in the medical and lay press, about this stress and strain, which was allegedly responsible for ulcers, coronaries and other maladies. As there is no means of measuring the stress and strain of life, objective evaluation of these ideas is impossible. But there seems absolutely no reason to suppose that people suffer more stress and strain now than they did in the past. In view of all our modern comforts and security the opposite seems more likely. In any case, we are not alone in believing that our age is more stressful than in the simple days of the past. Richard Asher[2] (1959) quotes the following passage from an address given in 1871 by Dr Crichton Browne: 'This is essentially a feverish and fidgety age, in which an unappeasable restlessness pervades all ranks and classes. The struggle for existence has become a melee and the recommendation to commune with your own heart in your chamber and be still is looked upon as an obsolete adage. The result of all this ceaseless agitation and ambitious striving is that the nervous system often gives way under the strain imposed on it. By a hideous kind of poetical justice, GPI has become a distorted reflection of the follies of the age. It is the miserable *otium cum dignitate* of the man of business'. It was not known in 1871 that GPI was due to syphilis.

The latest unifying theory is autoimmunity. Such maladies as rheumatoid arthritis, multiple sclerosis, and ulcerative colitis (which in the past were attributed to septic foci and later said to be psychosomatic) are now believed to be related to autoimmune mechanisms. There is indeed good evidence that such mechanisms are involved, but even if they are aetiological problems remain. We still have to explain why these mechanisms have begun to cause trouble to this particular individual at this particular time. We also still have to explain why one joint is destroyed by rheumatoid arthritis and another joint is spared.

Unifying theories also provide the basis to popular health cults. According to the age old Chinese practice of acupuncture ill health was believed to be due to an imbalance of the forces of *Yin*, the female element and *Yang*, the male element. And by inserting needles into certain points the equilibrium of *Yin* and *Yang* could be restored and the patient cured. Osteopathy depends on the theory that there is an 'osteopathic lesion' in the spine with all sorts of malign effects. Naturopathy depends on the theory that disease is due to 'unnatural' living habits, and that its cure is achieved by eating 'natural' foods and having such 'natural' remedies as colonic washouts. These cults are considered in Chapter 9.

There is no longer any wide acceptance in the medical world that there are single simple causes of pathological changes. We repeatedly read that conditions are multi-factorial. Coronary artery disease, for example, is said to be related to heredity, diet, the lack of exercise, smoking, and hypertension. We also read that the cause of various maladies is unknown. Thus, 'We still do not know what causes (hydronephrosis)'[3]. 'The aetiology of alopecia areata remains obscure'[4]. 'The exact cause of Raynaud's phenomenon is still unknown' (Goyle and Dormanby, 1976)[5]. 'The aetiology of Crohn's disease and of ulcerative colitis is obscure' (Cave and others, 1976)[6]. And so on.

Indeed, leaving aside injuries, the cause of all organic diseases is more or less obscure. We know that infections cannot occur if the necessary organism is absent, but we still have to explain why one person becomes ill with an infection and another person exposed to the same organism does not. We may answer this question by saying that the first person was susceptible to the infection and the second was not, but this leaves another unanswered question, 'What causes variations in susceptibility to infection?'. We know that a supremely important cause of squamous cell carcinoma of the bronchus is cigarette smoking, but this does not explain why seven out of eight of the heaviest smokers never develop cancer. And we also have to explain why people smoke heavily, knowing it to be harmful.

PSYCHOLOGICAL DISORDERS

Since psychological disorders are not, by definition, due to organic disease affecting the brain the possibility of making mistaken hypotheses about the aetiology of organic disease does not arise. But there have been theories that so-called psychological disorders are, in fact, due to brain disease. 'Neurasthenia', which was so common a label around the turn of this century, was attributed to fatigue of the nerve cells. As noted in Chapter 2, p. 25, during the First World War 'shell-shock' was attributed to widespread damage to the neurones from explosions. And there have been, and still are, suggestions that schizophrenia is 'really' organic, or is at least a biochemical disorder.

If the psychological disorders are considered solely on the psychological plane, there have been various theories to explain why people develop them. In the 19th century masturbation was widely believed to be an important cause, perhaps the most important cause, of insanity. In consequence, all sorts of barbaric practices were advocated to prevent it. John Hilton[7], in his celebrated book *Rest and Pain,* stated: (1863): 'I know of no way to prevent onanism except by freely blistering the penis, in order to make it raw and so sore that it cannot be touched without pain. This plan of treatment is sure to cure onanism'.

The most ambitious of the theories about the cause of psychological disorders is that of the analysts. This is considered in Chapter 9, p. 190 along with other cults.

Not only, then, must we give a most imperfect answer now to nearly all questions about aetiology. Whatever discoveries are made in the future, it is hardly conceivable that we shall ever be able to explain just why a particular individual develops a particular malady at a particular time. Whenever we succeed in answering one aetiological question there remains, and probably will always remain, another question which cannot be answered.

TREATMENT BASED ON THEORY

Provided no action is taken on account of mistaken theories of aetiology, no harm is done to the patient. The man who is thought to have fibrositis due to toxins from a septic focus suffers no damage if the doctor merely gives him a prescription for aspirin. But the main reason why we have made aetiological theories has been to discover remedies. And because many remedies have done so much harm, the supreme error of medicine throughout the ages has been to assume that treatment based either on theories of aetiology or on theories about the result of treatment *must* be effective.

The most ancient of all remedies of which we have solid information is trephining the skull, because trephined skulls thousands of years old have been discovered in various parts of the world. The reason for this remarkable procedure is thought to be that the subject was believed to be possessed by demons. A piece of skull was removed, to let the confined demons escape.

In the mid 19th century three widely used remedies were bleeding, starving, and purging. The theory behind bleeding was that the sick man's blood was believed to contain phlegma. This could be seen if his blood was allowed to stand; today he would be said to have a high ESR. As phlegma was evidently harmful, phlebotomy was clearly indicated. Fever had obvious similarities to a fire. Therefore, because a fire is put out by depriving it of fuel, a fever is damped down by depriving the patient of food. The bowel contents were responsible for intestinal auto-intoxication, with all sorts of noxious consequences. Who could doubt, therefore, that a purge should be given for almost every illness? And the fiercer the purge the more effective it was. Glauber's salts were good, but calomel and croton oil were even better.

In my student days bleeding was dead (except by some ophthalmologists, who applied leeches in treating inflammatory conditions affecting the eyes) and starving was only recommended for a few conditions such as bleeding peptic ulcer, though severely restricted diets were still popular in many circumstances. But purging was very much alive. The standard textbooks recommended a 'brisk purge' for all manner of conditions from eclampsia to febrile illnesses. Before nearly all operations patients were routinely given an enema. In Beaumont's *Medicine*[8] (1937 edition), a popular textbook of the time, we were informed that: 'In acute constipation happy results may follow the intramuscular injection of acetyl-choline, 0.1 g every 3 hours for 3 or 4 doses, when treatment by enemata or by croton oil has failed'. I do not recall croton oil being prescribed, though when I was working in a municipal hospital in Liverpool in 1935 every patient who was admitted to the unit for the mentally disordered was routinely given 3 grains of calomel. The theory behind this was, presumably, that by cleansing the bowels the brain would in turn be cleansed.

40 or 50 years ago vast numbers of luckless patients were given treatment depending on the septic focus theory. Their sinuses were washed out and their tonsils, appendices, and gall-bladders were removed. All this at least did no permanent harm, except when the patient died. But the most common method of eradicating septic foci was to remove teeth, and this might be followed by prolonged oral discomfort. Just after I qualified my mother complained that she was always hearing about the wonders of medicine but no-one did anything about the 'neuritis' affecting her right forearm. I therefore arranged for her to see an eminent neurologist, who took X-rays of her teeth, decided that the roots of some of her molars looked suspicious, and advised their removal. Her dentist did this unwillingly. She never got used to dentures for the rest of her life,

and she never ceased to regret the day when she went to Harley Street to see the eminent neurologist.

The theory that abdominal symptoms were due to ptosis led to some of the most appalling operations in the history of surgery. Pleats were taken in the stomach to cure gastroptosis and kidneys were hitched to the ribs to cure nephroptosis. Similarly, the round ligaments of the uterus were shortened to cure backache 'caused' by retroversion of the uterus.

In addition to the remedies based on theories of aetiology, there were many other remedies based on theories about the effect of treatment. Until recently an almost universal remedy was rest. It was indeed obvious to nearly everyone that rest must be beneficial to people with most illnesses. If patients with 'flu' and other febrile illnesses 'neglected' themselves by struggling on with their work their hearts would suffer damage or they would develop all sorts of complications. If people were so foolish as to get out of bed after abdominal operations their wounds would burst, their hearts would suffer, and various other disasters would happen. Healthy young men who had hernia repairs were therefore kept in bed for a few weeks.

Only a few years ago everyone knew that if a woman walked shortly after childbirth all sorts of complications would inevitably follow. In the 1969 edition of Holland and Brew's *Manual of Obstetrics*[9] we were told: 'If everyday activities are resumed when the uterus is as large as it is on the 10th day of the puerperium it is clear that there must be a liability to prolapse and subinvolution'. Indeed, so strong was the belief in the importance of rest in the puerperium that in 1953 the Ministry of Health issued the following edict: 'Maternity patients should not be discharged from hospital before the 10th day'. And in 1951 the report of the Central Midwives Board stated: 'In the case of training schools for pupil-midwives any system of discharge before the 10th day ... will cause the Board to reconsider the approval of the particular institution as a training school'. Here were examples of what has been considered the ultimate horror - the issuing of bureaucratic edicts telling doctors how to treat their patients. Yet these edicts did not produce a murmur of dissent.

30 or so years ago the unfortunate victim of ankylosing spondylitis would be encased in a plaster cast and kept on his back

for a year or more. In the days before streptomycin, PAS and isoniazid, bed rest was considered the supreme remedy for pulmonary tuberculosis and might be cöntinued for years. And some physicians at times prescribed 'absolute rest'. Even when the marvellous drugs became available prolonged rest continued to be advised for many years and to some extent it is still advised today.

Only 20 years ago nearly everyone took it for granted that rest was essential in treating patients who had suffered cardiac infarcts and for the first week or 2 many physicians regularly kept such patients at 'absolute rest'. The great Sir Thomas Lewis, by general acclaim the supreme scientific physician between the wars, made the following *ex cathedra* pronouncement in his *Diseases of the Heart* (1942 edition):[10] 'Rest in bed should be continued for from 6 to 8 weeks, to ensure firm cicatrization of the ventricular wall; during the whole of this period the patient is to be guarded by day and night nursing and helped in every way to avoid voluntary movement or effort'. Even after the 6 to 8 weeks the unfortunate patient would only be allowed to get about with extreme caution and not return to work for months, if then. The conscientious physician might well seek an interview with the victim's wife and explain to her that she held her husband's life in her hands and she should constantly guard him from worry and strain and ensure that he rested after each meal. The psychological state of both patient and wife, if they did as the doctors advised, can well be imagined.

20 or 30 years ago most patients were prescribed a modified diet. For a febrile illness the patient would perhaps be told to drink plentifully, avoid roast and fried foods and have dry toast, a lightly poached egg, beef tea, or grapes.

When the patient was affected by a disorder of the alimentary tract, there was particular emphasis on dieting. A striking example was the graduated diet for peptic ulcer, originally devised by Sippy and followed with modifications in all the standard medical text-books. All the large hospitals had their own diet sheets. The diet recommended in Beaumont's *Medicine*[8] (1937 edition) was as follows: Weeks 1 and 2: 5 ozs of citrated milk, flavoured with tea if desired, or Horlicks malted milk or Benger's food, every 2 hours. Week 3: Add one raw egg to two of the milk feeds. A little thin bread and butter is given with one feed and a little milk jelly or custard once daily. Week 4: The feeds are given every 2.5 hours and some include potato soup, cornflour, or sago pudding. Week 5: Pounded fish, lightly boiled egg, crisp toast or rusk (well chewed) with butter are added. Weeks 6 to 8: Minced meat is added. Then followed diet 2, for the convalescent stage of about a month. Such items as apple jelly, fresh white fish (boiled or steamed), rabbit, chicken or tender mutton, mashed potato, stewed apples (with no pips, skin, or core) are allowed. Thereafter, the patient would be advised diet 3, to be continued indefinitely. A fair variety is allowed, provided the food can be reduced to a soft pulp in the mouth and all meals are eaten slowly, well chewed and followed by rest for half an hour. But many items are forbidden permanently, including condiments, vinegar, smoked salmon, high game, sausages, curry, fried foods, all cheese except cream cheese, pickles, salads, uncooked vegetables, raw fruit, new or wholemeal bread, nuts, jam with pips, marmalade with peel, and alcohol. The reader of this astonishing passage could only assume that if minced meat is allowed in week 5 instead of week 6, or if the rusk is not well chewed, the healing of the ulcer will be delayed.

For patients with disorders of the colon, the traditional diet until recently was that it should be 'non-irritating' and low residue. Thus, according to *The Practice of Medicine*[11] (1956), '(Diverticulitis) usually settles with rest and reduction of colonic irritation by giving a low residue diet ... and advising liquid paraffin instead of aperients, without needing surgical intervention'. The foods to be avoided to ensure low residue were: '(1) Seeds, pips and skins in jam, fruit and tomatoes, (2) salads and whole vegetables, (3) nuts, coconut, dried fruit, candied peel, caraway seeds, angelica ..., (4) Shredded Wheat, All Bran, oatmeal, ginger and digestive biscuits, Ryvita and other crispbreads, 100% wholemeal bread and porridge, (5) spices, pepper (all kinds), mulligatawny, curry, vinegar, bottled sauces, pickles, chutney, mustard, onions and sausages'. A similar diet was advised for ulcerative colitis, 'mucous colitis' and 'irritable colon'.

The theory behind this dieting, both for peptic ulcer and for colonic conditions was, presumably, that it rested the diseased bowel. Taking only bland foods rested the stomach and low-residue foods rested the colon.

One of the commonest reasons for admission to a medical ward is drug overdosage. 20 years ago it was obvious that the correct treatment for hypnotic poisoning was an analeptic drug, since this clearly antagonized the hypnotic. Shulman and others[12] (1955), who were recognized authorities, stated that in cases of prolonged barbiturate coma, bemegride 'helps by bringing such a patient in 2 hours to a desired state of light anaesthesia'. And, according to a *Lancet* leading article[13] (1956) 'experienced clinicians believed that many of these patients (unconscious from barbiturates) would have died if bemegride had not been used.'

These various remedies based entirely on theory and all now derided are only the tip of the iceberg of medical folly. The list can be continued indefinitely. Among the other useless remedies based on theory are various diets (such as those to rest the kidneys or to rest the liver), depriving the victim of haematemesis of water, hot fomentations and poultices to draw out localized suppuration, heating the patient to overcome secondary 'shock', removing blood from the patient's arm and injecting it into his buttock (a form of 'non-specific protein therapy') to cure chronic or recurrent infection such as boils, gargles to cure sore throats, applying ichthyol to the skin or external ear to cure various inflammations, spa treatment, sea voyages, massage and a sojourn in places with 'relaxing' or 'bracing' climates.

The treatment sections of the standard textbooks of only 20 or 30 years ago were, indeed, largely uncritical rubbish - lists of recipes handed down from edition to edition and book to book. An extreme example is the following passage from Cecil's *Textbook of Medicine* (1943 edition), which was perhaps the most famous medical textbook of the time[14]. Patients with cerebral arteriosclerosis should (we were told) be treated thus: 'Avoidance of physical or mental over-exertion and the institution of rest-cures at home or in a sanatorium provide psychic rest and physical relaxation. Graduated exercises may be tried, but should be so regulated that the patient can rest for part of the day . . . Patients should be warned against straining at stool. Sexual activity must be limited . . . Excessive consumption of meat cannot be permitted. Curtailment of the salt intake is desirable. The meals ought to be small and taken with as little fluid as possible . . . The patient should reduce (weight) slightly. Alcohol, coffee and tobacco should be limited. Mineral oil or mild cathartics should be given to regulate the bowels. Warm baths and other forms of hydrotherapy are beneficial. "Nauheim" baths are also of service ... For the headache and vertigo ... hot fomentations may be applied to the forehead and neck. Mild massage is also of value. The high frequency current has its uses ... Iodides ... are said to delay the advance of the disease. Occasional doses of diuretics may be of service. Nitrites have been recommended to reduce hypertension'. This passage was removed entirely in the subsequent edition.

THE SITUATION TODAY

All the remedies mentioned in the last section are now dead or dying. Patients with some of the maladies for which these remedies were given are now given treatment with the opposite effect. Those with diverticular disease, for example, are advised diets containing a high residue and the victims of cardiac infarction are, at least after the first few weeks, encouraged to take vigorous exercise. Leaving aside gluten enteropathy, diabetes, obesity, and anorexia nervosa diets have been largely debunked, and within wide limits patients are encouraged to eat what they like.

The doctors of the past were not more stupid than are the doctors of today. Why, then, did we continue to use these remedies, now agreed to be useless or harmful, for all these years? Why should *a priori* reasoning that they were beneficial have been stronger than empirical evidence that they were not?

The main explanation is that nearly all the maladies for which these remedies were advised were either acute or recurrent disorders. Patients recover or improve from these maladies by the aid of nature alone. It was taken for granted that the recovery or improvement had been due to the remedy, when in fact it was due to nature. We made, indeed, one of the historic errors of reasoning; we fell into the trap of the *post hoc ergo propter hoc* fallacy (afterwards, therefore because of). Most doctors waited until controlled trials had been carried out, in which alternate patients were given, and alternate patients were denied some remedy, until they were persuaded to discard the remedy in question. And even then, many did so only gradually and reluctantly.

Ankylosing spondylitis provides an exception to the rule that conditions for which useless or harmful treatment was advised were either acute or recurrent. It is infinitely variable in severity but tends to be slowly progressive. Here, the orthopaedic surgeon who advised immobilization of the patient in a plaster cast for a year or so would be able to convince himself at the end of this period that if the patient had not been immobilized he would have become much worse. He, too, was seduced by the *post hoc ergo propter hoc* fallacy.

For reasons which are not clear to me we were more easily persuaded to stop using useless drugs than we were to stop using useless (or harmful) regimes and diets. Yet most of the traditional drugs were fairly harmless, whereas useless regimes or diets often had appalling effects. To develop ankylosing spondylitis is itself a most unpleasant fate; when in addition the wretched victim is encased in a plaster jacket for a year or so his fate does not bear thinking about, especially as he ended up more disabled than he would have been if he had escaped medical attention. For most people eating is one of the pleasures of life. To live for the rest of one's life deprived of condiments, vinegar, smoked salmon, high game, sausages, curry, fried foods, all cheese except cream cheese, pickles, salads, uncooked vegetables, raw fruits, new or wholemeal bread, jam with pips, marmalade with peel, and alcohol, as those with peptic ulcer were advised to do, is a grim prospect indeed. No doubt most of those given this advice ignored it, but this does not make the advice any less awful.

The earlier controlled trials were, then, all of drugs, or possibly of operations, but not of rest, diet, climatotherapy, physiotherapy, manipulation, speech therapy, etc. Indeed, to this day there have been few trials of these general measures. One of the best known of the early trials was of the streptomycin treatment of tuberculosis. This was conducted by a committee of the Medical Research Council and in the paper giving the result of the trial it was stated[15] (1948): 'The natural course of pulmonary tuberculosis is in fact so variable and unpredictable that evidence of improvement or cure following the use of a new drug cannot be accepted as proof of the effect of that drug ... It had become obvious that, in future, conclusions regarding the clinical effect of a new chemotherapeutic agent in tuberculosis could be considered valid only if based on adequately controlled clinical trials ... Determination of whether a patient would be treated by streptomycin and bed-rest (s case) or by bed-rest alone (c case) was made by reference to a statistical series based on random sampling numbers by Prof. Bradford Hill; the details of the series were unknown to any of the investigators or to the co-ordinator and were contained in a set of sealed envelopes, each bearing on the outside only the name of the hospital and number'. But all patients were treated by bed rest. The Medical Research Committee did not say: 'it is obvious that conclusions regarding rest in tuberculosis can be considered valid only if based on adequately controlled clinical trials'. And even after that most spectacularly successful of all curative treatment, the combination of streptomycin, PAS and ixoniazid, had been in general use for years most patients were kept in bed as well. We shall never know whether rest, which was widely believed to be the supremely important treatment for tuberculosis in the prechemotherapeutic era, had in the long term any beneficial effect at all.

In spite of all the work by Sir A. Bradford Hill, Sir Richard Doll and others in carrying out trials, to this day we still give many remedies of unproven value, solely for theoretical reasons. One explanation is inertia. Even when remedies have been effectively debunked, they are still used and still sometimes recommended in recent articles.

When I was a medical student the 'fat-free' diet for infective hepatitis was already being derided by the forward thinkers. Indeed, if the matter is looked at from a theoretical angle it is most difficult to understand why the presence of imperfectly digested fat in the intestine should damage the liver. When I had the condition myself in India in 1943 I was ordered a fat-free diet as a patient in my own military hospital. As I objected to eating dry bread I waited until the ward-sister was at lunch and would then nip out of bed and steal some butter from the ward-kitchen. I was once caught in the act and soundly ticked off by the ward-sister who told me that I ought to know better. As recently as 1976 I was asked to see a jaundiced patient in a surgical ward. Noting that he was on a fat-free diet I asked the house surgeon why this was so and was told that most jaundiced people do not like fat. I replied that if the patient did not like fat he wouldn't eat it, but asked why should he be served dry bread if he wanted to have some butter with it? To this question the house surgeon made no answer but looked most uncomfortable. Around the same time a patient who had been under my care with infective hepatitis asked me when she attended the out-patient department how long she must continue with a fat-free diet. For, in spite of my repeated insistence that patients with hepatitis could eat what they wanted, a ward-sister, knowing that of course jaundiced people do not eat fat, had given her a fat-free diet sheet on discharge.

Even more surprising, modified diet and other unsupported treatment is still advised in recent articles. Thus Read[16] (1975) says: 'Infective hepatitis due to hepatitis virus A infection is usually a self-limiting disorder which responds to bed rest, nursing and dietary treatment'. The 'dietary treatment' is not specified, but this passage clearly implies that if a patient gets out of bed if he feels so inclined, is not nursed, and eats what he fancies, his recovery will be impaired. Murray-Lyon and Reynolds [17] (1976), writing in the *'Today's Treatment'* series, likewise say: 'The mainstay of treatment for infectious hepatitis remains a nutritious diet and bed rest, though various clinical trials have failed to show that bed rest is beneficial'. This one sentence illustrates how slowly old ideas may die. For, although there is no evidence from trials that bed rest is beneficial, it is still said to be the 'mainstay of treatment'. And no evidence is advanced that a 'nutritious diet' makes any difference.

Patients with infective hepatitis are customarily told to have no alcohol for from 3 to 6 months. This depends on the theory that infective hepatitis is a disease of the liver, alcohol damages the liver and therefore the patient with infective hepatitis should have no alcohol. Murray-Lyon and Reynolds[17] (1976) say: 'During the recovery phase the traditional 3 to 6 month's embargo on alcohol remains in vogue'. What we wish to know is whether or not patients with hepatitis who drink alcohol fare worse than those who do not. Apparently, no clinical trials have been performed to determine this. No doubt the safest advice is to tell patients to keep off alcohol, as this cannot do them harm and may do them good. But authors should at least point out that the embargo on alcohol is advised solely for theoretical reasons, evidence being unavailable.

Patients with gall-bladder disease are likewise still told to keep off fats and eggs. Indeed, the knowledgeable public 'know' that this is so. This also is derived wholly from theory; there is no evidence that eating fats or eggs does any harm.

The low-residue diet for diverticular disease and other disorders of the colon has disappeared without trace. But patients with peptic ulcer may still be advised a modified diet over and above the commonsense advice that they should avoid anything which they find from experience is upsetting. They may be told to avoid fried and roast foods and 'irritants' such as pepper, mustard and vinegar, or be merely urged to 'eat sensibly', whatever that may mean.

In spite of all the debunking of rest during recent years many doctors still advise rest in many situations almost as a reflex action. And rest is still advocated in the very latest articles solely for theoretical reasons, in circumstances when there is no evidence that it is beneficial. I have already noted above that the subjects of pulmonary tuberculosis and infective hepatitis are still advised to rest. Patients who have suffered a subarachnoid haemorrhage are often kept strictly in bed for 6 weeks, though no evidence has been advanced that those who do so fare better than those who do not. No doubt many doctors take the view that rest is so obviously essential after a subarachnoid haemorrhage that it would be unethical to carry out a controlled trial in which alternate patients are allowed to get up. I do not accept that this argument is valid, but even if it is assumed that patients should be rested, why should 6 weeks be the correct figure? It could hardly be maintained that it would be unethical to rest alternate patients for 6 weeks and the others for 4 weeks. If it were found that those who rested for 4 weeks did just as well as those who rested for 6 weeks, further trials could compare 4 weeks rest with 2 weeks rest and finally 2 weeks rest with no rest.

In my student days a condition for which rest was advocated with especial fervour was rheumatic fever. For as this often involves the heart, it was obvious to everyone that to minimize the damage prolonged rest, up to many months, was essential. Controlled trials to determine whether rest does in fact do good have not been done. St. John Sutton and Rubenstein[18] (1974) analysed a multicentre controlled co-operative trial in 1955 to assess the efficacy of aspirin, cortisone and ACTH. They observed that in 1961 Bywaters and Thomas compared the effect of 6 weeks bed rest alone, bed rest plus salicylates and bed rest plus steroids. The one remedy they do not analyse is bed rest. They merely state: 'Bed rest ... remains an essential part of treatment'. Why should bed rest be immune from criticism?

It is taken for granted that hypertensive pregnant women should be rested and sedated. The theoretical edifice behind this practice is obvious: hypertension is associated with toxaemia and foetal loss; bed rest and sedation lower the blood pressure; therefore bed rest and sedation will lower the incidence of toxaemia and foetal loss. In addition, it has been claimed that placental circulation is lessened by exercise, which gives a further theoretical basis to rest. Nevertheless, there is no evidence from clinical trials that rest is beneficial. Matthews[19] (1977) conducted a randomized controlled trial of 135 patients designed to determine whether bed rest and sedation are of any general benefit to either the mother or the baby in pregnancies complicated by mild non-albuminuric and asymptomatic hypertension after the 28th week. The results suggested that neither mother nor babies benefited. Yet large numbers of beds in obstetric departments are occupied by non-albuminuric, asymptomatic, hypertensive, pregnant women.

Even though actual bed rest is now advocated uncommonly, patients are still often advised to take lesser degrees of rest. They may be urged, for example, not to 'overdo it' or to 'take things easily'. And even when the doctor does not give such advice the patient himself, or perhaps more often his spouse, may take it for granted that obviously it must be bad to engage in vigorous exercise. This especially applies to men with coronary artery disease or after operations. For when we doctors have repeatedly told the public for generations that people who have had heart attacks should rest completely for weeks and not overdo it for life, it is hardly surprising that the public should still retain these beliefs, although most of us have now changed our attitude.

A type of dieting which remains widely popular is that designed to lessen the likelihood of coronary artery disease. Huge numbers of people throughout the affluent world, especially in the United States, now eat sparingly of animal fat with this end in view. Few subjects have stimulated such a spate of articles in recent years as has this. The theoretical basis to this kind of dieting is evident. People with a high level of cholesterol and other lipids in their blood have an increased liability to coronary artery disease. A diet low in saturated fat lowers the blood level of these lipids. Therefore, this diet will lower the incidence of coronary artery disease. Here, we do not have to depend solely on theory, as large numbers of trials have been carried out. There has been endless debate on this matter and conflicting interpretations have been made of the trials. However, there is no unequivocal evidence that this kind of dieting does in fact lower the incidence of coronary artery disease. McMichael[20] (1979), recently Professor of Medicine at the Royal Post Graduate Medical School of London, comments: 'All well controlled trials of cholesterol-reducing diets and drugs have failed to reduce coronary mortality and morbidity'.

Similar considerations apply to the drug clofibrate, which has been prescribed for vast numbers of men for many years because of its cholesterol-lowering effect. A recent trial[21] (1978) of over 10 000 people with elevated blood cholesterol levels indicated that clofibrate had no effect on the mortality from coronary heart disease (and the incidence of gall-stones requiring surgery was significantly higher in those given clofibrate).

Throughout my career I never advised a modified diet (other than a low calorie diet for the obese) or prescribed clofibrate for patients with coronary artery disease. I maintained throughout that these treatments were given for theoretical reasons and that I intended to wait until there was evidence that they were effective before I subjected unfortunate patients to them.

On p. 147 I noted that 20 years ago patients poisoned by hypnotic drugs were given analeptics on theoretical grounds. It is now agreed that this treatment was positively harmful. Among 100 patients poisoned by hypnotics who are admitted alive to hospital, we know that if no treatment is given, some 90 to 95 or even more will recover. We also know that one or two have taken so large a dose that no treatment will save them. Therefore, treatment can only matter to at most some three or four of these patients. This is the archetypal situation which can only be resolved by a clinical trial. And a very large-scale trial is needed to obtain a result. Unfortunately there has been a singular lack of such trials. Theory, therefore, still reigns supreme here.

Trials are not needed to determine that certain kinds of treatment should be given to patients unconscious from drugs. If the patient's airway is blocked, steps should be taken to keep it unblocked. The patient's position should be changed, since we can be sure that this will make pressure sores less likely. And if he remains unconscious for long he should be given fluid, either by intragastric or intravenous tube. Indeed, in most situations the latest articles on this matter advise that only this kind of supportive treatment is needed. But in certain situations other more vigorous measures are advocated. Thus, Matthew and Lawson[22] (1975) in *Treatment of Common Acute Poisonings* - widely used as a reference book by casualty officers - state that when the plasma salicylate concentration exceeds 500 mg intensive forced diuretic treatment must be started. They also advocate eliminative measures for severe lithium, meprobamate, chloral, primidone, barbiturate and phenobarbitone poisoning. Lawson (1976) also states[23]: 'There is no doubt that there are instances when these measures of elimination are extremely valuable and may be life-saving'. Vale[24] (1978), dealing with paediatric poisoning, likewise lays down that if the plasma salicylate concentration exceeds 500 mg per litre, forced alkaline diuresis should be instituted.

These eliminative measures are advised because some of the poison is thereby removed from the body. Theory, therefore, indicates that the procedure is beneficial. But there is no proof that in consequence the patient's life will be saved. And saving life, not removing poison, is the object of the exercise. I have twice pointed this out[25,26] in the medical press (Todd, 1973 and 1978) but on neither occasion did the protagonists of eliminative treatment reply. The doctors who actually deal with poisoned patients are the juniors in hospitals. As they are told by the Authorities that they *must* carry out eliminative treatment in certain circumstances they will naturally assume that this is of proven value. The Authorities should at least make it clear that their advice is based on theory, not on evidence. If eliminative treatment were harmless, one could argue that it should be given, even in the absence of evidence that it is effective. But, as everyone knows, it is positively dangerous, and many patients have been killed by it.

Poisoned patients are also given other treatment for theoretical reasons. According to Matthew[27] (1968): 'If raising the foot of the bed is not sufficient to raise the (systolic) pressure (of poisoned patients) to 100 mmHg, metaraminol 5 mg intramuscularly may be injected and repeated 20 minutes later if required. If two doses of 5 mg metaraminol at an interval of 20 minutes fail to produce the necessary rise in blood pressure, plasma expanders should be used without delay'. Once more, there is no evidence that these measures save lives. Moreover, metaraminol was widely used a few years ago to raise the blood pressure of patients with cardiogenic shock, but it is now generally thought that this actually worsened the prognosis.

In Chapter 5, p. 93, when dealing with High Technology medicine I noted that in Intensive Care Units patients are closely monitored and if abnormalities are found, these are regularly corrected. If there is acidosis, lactate or bicarbonate are added to the drip; if there is alkalosis, ammonium chloride is given instead. In the serum potassium is low, potassium chloride is added to the drip; if it is high, an ion exchange resin is given. If the haemoglobin is below a certain level, a blood transfusion is given; if it is above another level, venesection is performed. If there are ectopic beats, lignocaine is added to the drip; if there is 2:1 block atropine is given. All these things are done for theoretical reason. Possibly some of them sometimes save life, but it should not be taken for granted that 'correcting' some parameter will save life. We can only find actual evidence by comparing similar patients who are given some particular treatment with others who are denied it.

We regularly read about 'rational' treatment, which is the antithesis of 'empirical' treatment. Thus in a *British Medical Journal* leading article[28] (1979), we read: 'perhaps the most important thing for us to realize is that, after countless years of empiricism, the controlled trial has emerged as a sharp tool for dissection of certain problems ... Some guidelines are visible: when there is no rational or *a priori* basis for preferring one treatment to another the prospective controlled trial is wholly appropriate'. In another *British Medical Journal* leading article[29] (1979) we are told: 'once we understand the pathogenesis of alopecia areata we may hope to devise rational treatment. Meanwhile effective empirical treatments may provide useful clues to the nature of the disease'.

Rational treatment is, therefore, said to be treatment devised by *a priori* reasoning. Empirical means 'based on, or guided by, the results of observation and experiment only'. A controlled trial is, in fact, an example of empirical experiment. Unfortunately, medical writers habitually say *empirical* when they mean its antithesis *theoretical*. We did not have 'countless years of empiricism', as we were told in the *British Medical Journal* leading article mentioned above; we had countless years of devising treatment from theory. The only rational ground I know for giving treatment is the existence of empirical evidence that it is effective.

In spite, then, of the profound change in medical attitudes which has accompanied the widespread realization that controlled clinical trials are often needed to evaluate treatment, there still remains this strong attachment to *a priori* reasoning. Many traditional remedies continue to be used, although there is no evidence that they do good. Many remedies derived from theory, such as eliminative treatment for poisoning and clofibrate to reduce the incidence of coronary artery disease, have only been devised in recent years. Yet no evidence is forthcoming that they are effective. And medical writers habitually refer to rational treatment, by which they mean treatment based on theory.

Clear-cut evidence about the value of many remedies does not exist, so when considering whether or not to use them we are compelled to rely on theory. But those who teach and write should at least distinguish between theory and practice. And this is what so many lamentably fail to do. No doubt one reason for this failure is that the writer just does not realize that some remedy which he states is 'life-saving' is of unproven value. It may seem obvious, for example, that as forced alkaline diuresis removes some salicylate from the body it *must* be the right treatment. It is forgotten that the object of the treatment is to save the patient's life, and there is no proof that forced alkaline diuresis does so.

When from lack of evidence we are compelled to depend on theory the burden of proof should, then, be made to rest on those who advocate, not on those who oppose, some remedy. In the past this burden was made to rest on the opponents of treatment. Bleeding, starving, purging, resting etc., continued to be used until daring sceptics stopped prescribing them and persuaded their orthodox and unthinking colleagues that patients thereby did better. If only our predecessors had stopped using all those useless and harmful remedies because they were based on theory and of unproven value, how different would medical history have been!

FORGETTING THE PATIENT

The third great error of medicine is to forget the patient. I have referred to this repeatedly throughout this book, especially in Chapters 2, 3 and 7. Extreme examples of this error occurred in the teaching hospitals when I was a student. Some of the great men then considered patients to be clinical material possessing physical signs for the education and edification of the students. And sometimes the patient's problems would be discussed in his hearing, just as if he was a dog being taken to the vet.

This error has little relevance to patients with acute disasters. When someone has a massive cardiac infarct, meningitis, fractured femur, haematemesis, diabetic ketosis, or an 'acute abdomen' the doctor should rightly concentrate on the malady and pay little attention to the patient (apart from remembering to speak kindly to him and to relieve his pain). And when there is some gross organic lesion, especially if progressive, such as malignant disease, ankylosing spondylitis, or Parkinson's disease, a large part of the attention should be devoted to the disease. But such maladies have grave emotional repercussions and, although the doctor cannot do a great deal to help, he should constantly bear this in mind and try to minimize the patient's distress.

The error of forgetting the patient is disastrous when patients have long-standing somatic symptoms, whether or not these are related to some chronic benign lesion or are 'functional' (using functional in the sense defined in Chapter 3, p. 43) or psychosomatic. Patients of this kind provide a large proportion of those referred to hospitals as out-patients, and especially to physicians.

Many patients with long-standing symptoms were given the bogus diagnoses and prescribed the mistaken remedies described in the first two sections of this chapter. If those surgeons who diagnosed visceroptosis or intestinal auto-intoxication (and then pleated stomachs and removed colons) had not concentrated all their attention on patient's bellies but had sat back and looked at them as people, they would not have made these awful errors. For it would then have been obvious that these patients were chronically unwell, depressed or worried people, perhaps living wholly unsatisfactory lives, with multiple somatic symptoms, as well as their abdominal symptoms.

Forgetting the patient has been the particular error of the consultant rather than the GP. Even if the GP takes a mechanistic view of patients' symptoms, he can hardly be unaware of their circumstances. He knows, for example, that a woman with long-standing abdominal discomfort, 'wind', nausea and constipation lives a most unhappy life with a brutal alcoholic husband and that at other times she has attended with headache, backache, weakness, tiredness and other symptoms.

Consultants are less mechanistic and narrow in their attitude today than were their predecessors. Physicians at least mostly try to look at the patient as well as his presenting symptoms. But, it is to be feared, many of the ultra-specialists still take the view that their business is to deal only with the organ or region in which they specialize. If a patient with headache is sent to the ENT surgeon to 'exclude an ENT cause' the surgeon may do just this. If in fact the ear, nose, and throat are found normal, no great harm results. Mistakes are made when some abnormality, such as an opaque sinus to X-ray or a deflected nasal septum, are found. Far too often the surgeon takes it for granted that the abnormality is the cause of the headache. Whereas if he acted as a consultant, not as a specialist, it would perhaps be obvious that the kind of long-standing headache of which the patient complains could not be due to sinusitis or a deflected nasal septum.

Some ultra-specialists, indeed, appear to wear blinkers by choice. The ophthalmologist may look at humanity solely through his lenses and his ophthalmoscope. The ENT surgeon takes the patient into a dark room to transilluminate his sinuses and insert his laryngoscope and then studies his X-rays. The rectal specialist's field of vision may be limited to what he can see through his sigmoidoscope, and the gynaecologist studies his patients through the vaginal speculum.

A condition of which much has been written during the last 25 years is the Munchausen syndrome - a term coined[30] by Richard Asher (1951). All doctors who have worked in hospitals, especially in large cities, are familiar with the subjects of the syndrome, who are repeatedly admitted to hospital with fake symptoms of various kinds, such as severe chest pain, severe bellyache suggesting an acute abdomen, severe headache, 'collapse', and bleeding from the mouth or ears. Perhaps the most extravagant example of the syndrome was described by Pallis and Bambi[31] (1979). The story of the man concerned began with several admissions to the City Hospital, Belfast, in 1944 with a knee injury that failed to heal. In 1947 he was transferred from a Belfast Prison to a mental hospital, where he spent 5 years. Between 1954 and 1976 he was admitted innumerable times to many London, English provincial, and Belfast hospitals. He had recurrent episodes of headache, photophobia, neck stiffness and left hemiplegia. Subarachnoid haemorrhage was repeatedly diagnosed, but numerous lumbar punctures yielded clear fluid. Many carotid angiograms were performed, all normal. He often demanded large doses of analgesics. In 1961 after several episodes of dysphagia, dysphonia, and 'acute respiratory failure' (for which emergency tracheostomy was performed) he acquired a permanent tracheostomy, probably in Doncaster. In 1965 he began to complain of abdominal pain. Dozens of barium swallows, meals and enemas and at least four laparotomies were performed. He had numerous emergency admissions for chest pain, with or without episodes of hemiparesis, as well as for acute abdominal pain. In 1975 after an admission for chest pain he developed acute retention of urine and transurethral prostatectomy was performed. In 1976 he was admitted to the City Hospital, Belfast, with a fractured right femur. Pinning was unsuccessful and he later underwent total hip replacement at St. Mary's Hospital, London. Pallis and Bambi documented 207 admissions (though without doubt there were many more than this) and commented: 'All of his acute symptoms and signs were faked, with the exception of his fractured femur and the possible exception of his retention of urine'.

Some doctors have said that they cannot be blamed for having been taken in by the subjects of the Munchausen syndrome, for we must assume that when patients complain of some symptom they are telling the truth. But if only the doctor does not just concentrate all his attention on the particular region from which the symptom arises but sits back and looks at the man as a whole, the diagnosis of the Munchausen syndrome becomes as a rule one of the simplest of all to reach. And no-one can pretend that this syndrome is so rare that one can be excused for overlooking it; every doctor has heard of it and the diagnosis is often made by a hospital porter, who has seen the subject many times before. Often I have been able to reach the diagnosis with absolute confidence just by a description over the telephone. I recall several patients with the following kind of story. The house physician has rung me to say that he is worried about an emergency admission who is, say, bleeding from the mouth and appears to be in agonizing chest pain. I have inquired how was the patient admitted and where did he live, which the HP did not know. Later the HP has rung back to say that the man says he lives in Glasgow and got off a bus or train because he felt so ill and was brought to the hospital by the police. I then asked why he was in Farnham, Surrey, to be informed later that he stated he was on his way to, say, Southampton, to get a job. Frequently, the patient would become increasingly indignant as this kind of inquiry was made and flaws in his story were pointed out, and he might well say he was better and walk out of the hospital. I used to tell my juniors that anyone who gave a remote address and was alleged to be taken ill in the street was highly likely to be an example of the Munchausen syndrome. If, in addition, the patient did not, as would those who were not faking their symptoms, urge that his relatives be informed of his illness, the diagnosis was even more probable. Another fruitful line of inquiry was to ask the name of the patient's doctor. Sometimes he would say that he had no doctor or could not remember his name, and if he gave a name and address no such person could usually be found in the *Medical Directory*. Many of the less extravagant examples of the syndrome wanted no more than a night's rest with supper and breakfast and early the following morning would insist that they were better and walk out of the hospital, sometimes being made to sign a form that they were discharging themselves against medical advice!

The manner in which these numerous people with the Munchausen syndrome are so often mishandled in hospital is, indeed, a grave reflection on our clinical acumen and a striking example of the error of failing to look at the patient as a whole. All these repeated expensive investigations and repeated laparotomies provide a dismal testimony of our folly. The excuse is sometimes made that the Munchausen syndrome was, indeed, suspected but that it would be 'unfair' to the patient to assume that he must be a liar, so to be on the safe side various investigations were done to 'exclude organic disease'. This is one more example of the absurd error of diagnosing neurosis by exclusion (see Chapter 3, p. 38). It is also said sometimes that these unfortunate people are sick and should be given treatment.No doubt they are mentally sick, but there is no evidence that treatment is effective. In particular, doing vast numbers of investigations and keeping them in hospital for weeks at enormous expense makes them worse, not better.

Although there would be widespread agreement with the view that, especially when dealing with chronic complainers, the doctor should look at the patient as a whole, not just at his presenting symptoms, there is also opposition to this approach. Thus, Dornhorst and Hunter[32] (1967) say: 'The pastoral fallacy is a creation of a section of the profession and probably arises as a reaction by those no longer able to keep abreast with the technical complexities of modern medicine. Its proponents emphasize the distinction between the patient and his disease and claim to treat the whole man and to regard the patient as a person. They stress the frequency and educational importance of the more trivial disorders and their interrelation with emotional factors. There is an implication that much of the elaboration of modern investigation and treatment could be dispensed with if doctors were trained to acquire wisdom rather than to accumulate technical knowledge. Pervaded by an excessive belief in the unique therapeutic relation between doctor and patient, they aim to substitute a pastoral role for technical care, which is assumed to be necessarily impersonal and even inhumane. This approach is often sympathetically received by laymen who are alarmed by various features of modern life, from divorce rates to sonic booms. They believe that all would be well if doctors would turn their attention to prevention rather than cure and that medical students should learn more about health than about disease. The fallacy is a favourite with the amateur psycho-analysts who figure so prominently in left-wing journalism and is also supported, for opportunist reasons, by some professional specialties and by all manner of cranks and faddists. The essential superficiality, and indeed dishonesty, of this attitude is revealed when one of its advocates is faced with illness in himself or in his family. The call then is not for the wise father figure, but for the man who knows most about so and so'.

If Dornhorst and Hunter had said that they were considering only patients who needed surgery, or had severe acute illnesses, their approach could be defended. The patient with an 'acute abdomen' does not need careful appraisal of his emotional background; he should be seen by a surgeon who has all modern technical aids to help him. But the overwhelming majority of patients have some minor self-limiting ailment, some chronic condition for which there is no radical treatment, or are emotionally disturbed. Who knows most about those numerous patients who complain of persistent dull headache, muzziness, chronic low backache, weakness, exhaustion, being 'always tired', 'wind', 'catarrh', aching in the limbs, constipation etc? Who is most likely to select correctly the very few who should be investigated from the vast majority who should not? If there is a question of operation for a chronic benign condition, such as varicose veins, gastric ulcer, gall-bladder disease, or menorrhagia, which surgeon will make the wisest decision? The doctor who can see the patient as a whole and who looks into his background and relationships, not the one who knows most about so and so, can best deal with all such patients.

OVER-VALUING TECHNOLOGY

All three errors so far discussed have a very long history. And they are all made less often than in the past. Erroneous theories of aetiology are now rarely made by doctors, though they remain the stock-in-trade of the followers of cults. Treatment devised solely from theory, and of unproven value, is still given, but far less than it was. And there is at least considerable acceptance of the idea that the patient as a whole, not just the region of his presenting complaint, should be looked at.

The great modern error is the over-valuation of technology. Of course technology plays an essential part in the spectacular triumphs of medicine. All surgery and anaesthetics are dependent on technology. X-rays, computer-assisted tomography, all kinds of scopes and other means of diagnosis can be of great practical value. All the successes of modern treatment, such as the antibiotics and hormones, depend on technology for their discovery and manufacture, however simple is their actual administration. But in only a tiny minority of all clinical situations is technology relevant. Our error lies in using it inappropriately and attaching too much importance to it.

The abuse of technology is mainly considered in Chapter 5. Here, I describe the grossly excessive investigations throughout the Western world, and in particular the absurd practice of doing vast numbers of routine investigations on everyone. I also consider the unwise surgery, the over-zealous use of radiotherapy, cancer chemotherapy, blood transfusions and other kinds of intravenous therapy and much of what happens in Intensive Care Units. Especially when dealing with very ill patients it is easy to assume that the more that is done the better. If a patient has assisted respiration, tracheostomy, continuous oxygen and a drip into each arm (into one of which is going blood and the other various drugs), along with the monitoring of all parameters the physician can solace himself when the patient dies that everything possible has been done. And even if the physician has his doubts, the relatives will take it for granted that the finest scientific medicine has been used.

To a large extent, indeed, high technology medicine is wrongly equated with medicine of a high standard. And in the last few years in Britain one has hardly been able to open a medical journal or a newspaper without reading of falling medical standards. High dignitaries of the medical profession regularly issue solemn warnings on this topic. A characteristic example appeared in a *Times* leading article (July 12, 1978) in which the Chairman of the British Medical Association, Dr James Cameron, was reported as saying that 'standards were rapidly deteriorating in the NHS'.

But on the great majority of occasions when a patient seeks medical advice high technology should play no part. The patient should have no investigations, no hospital referral, and no prescription (apart possibly from an analgesic). The GP who does just this achieves the highest possible standard of medical care. By contrast, his colleague who orders a series of futile investigations, gives a variety of fatuous prescriptions (including perhaps a benzodiazepine, an anorectic, vitamins, a tonic and a so-called peripheral vasodilator) and refers the patient, for no other reason than that the patient demands it, to a consultant (who admits the patient to hospital where he has another long series of futile investigations followed by an unnecessary operation) achieves an abysmally low standard of care.

There is a widespread tendency to take it for granted that a result in concrete terms emanating from a laboratory or an X-ray department represents Truth, whereas the clinical picture, and especially the symptoms, are essentially subjective and therefore of little value. The reason why the patient seeks medical advice is that he has symptoms and it is the doctor's business to relieve these symptoms. Sometimes this is best achieved just by giving a symptomatic drug; at other times it may be possible to discover with the aid of sophisticated investigations some condition which can be cured by advanced surgery. The decision as to which course is right can only be taken by the doctor after assessing the symptoms and assessing the patient against his background.

In any case, the diagnosis must often be reached just from the symptoms. No advanced technology can determine whether or not someone has migraine or dysmenorrhoea. If a patient complains of pain in the calf which regularly comes on after he has walked a certain distance, this provides sufficient evidence that the arterial circulation to his leg is impaired. There may be associated findings, such as an absent femoral pulse or an obstructed artery on the arteriogram, but these do not in themselves prove that impaired circulation is the cause of the pain. When someone has recurrent chest pain there may be uncertainty as to whether this is due to myocardial ischaemia. If the e.c.g. is abnormal this will suggest that myocardial ischaemia is probably responsible. But an abnormal e.c.g. does not prove that chest pain must be due to the heart. Whereas if someone gives a history that he regularly develops praecordial pain after walking a certain distance, which is soon relieved by rest, and that on a cold day or after a meal the pain develops sooner and that if he takes TNT before setting off the pain comes on after a longer distance, we have the best of all evidence of myocardial ischaemia (provided the patient is not telling lies).

During my Army career in the War many directives stated or implied that malaria can be diagnosed only by finding the parasite in the blood. But if a patient had rigors and high fever on alternate days any other cause but malaria was most unlikely. The finding of parasites in people who have had malaria throughout their lives does not prove that their present illness is due to malaria. And the failure to find parasites in people who had just been infected for the first time does not prove that their fever is non-malarial. If some expert spends hours in studying a series of blood samples, perhaps he can always find a few parasites when a patient is in fact ill from malaria. But such experts with hours of time to spare did not exist in the Army during the War.

Previously in this chapter (p. 137) I discussed the error of wrongly relating symptoms to some abnormality (such as retroversion of the uterus or astigmatism) which happened to be present. Technology has greatly increased the opportunities of making this kind of error. Pathogenic organisms may be found which are doing no harm but to which an illness is wrongly attributed. Patients may be wrongly diagnosed as thyrotoxic because the tests are outside some arbitrary range. Backache is wrongly attributed to 'arthritis of the spine' on account of X-ray changes. And dyspepsia is wrongly attributed to gall-bladder disease because gall-stones are seen on the X-ray. Indeed, each new technological advance tends to be followed by a spate of erroneous diagnoses. In my student days the diagnosis of 'gastritis' in patients with dyspepsia was derided in my medical school because there was no proof that the symptoms were due to gastritis. Then around 1937 the flexible gastroscope became available and many bright young registrars were learning to use this marvellous new tool. In consequence, numerous dyspeptics were said to have 'chronic hypertrophic gastritis'. Within a few years it was realized that the gastroscopic appearances were unrelated to the symptoms and the diagnosis of gastritis disappeared once more.

Even those who are willing to accept the fallibility of X-rays, e.c.g.s and other investigations may nevertheless cling to the belief that one particular procedure, namely histology, really is infallible. How often do we read the term 'histologically proved'!

In many circumstances histology can provide unequivocal evidence. When a patient has enlarged cervical glands which could be tuberculous or malignant, the histologist can give a clear-cut answer. But in other circumstances histology can be misleading, for several reasons.

(1) A 'histologically proved' lesion which is said to be present is in fact present, but this is not the cause of the patient's symptoms.

(2) Biopsy specimens may be taken, say from the liver or kidney, which are rightly reported as normal, although these organs are in fact affected by disseminated disease with interspersed normal areas. Histology, like other means of investigation, often cannot exclude some suspected condition.

(3) In practice some sections are difficult to interpret and the best

of all histologists cannot give a confident opinion. Less than perfect histologists may make the all too human error of making a confident statement on insufficient grounds. Great though the value of histology is in many circumstances it has, like other means of investigation, strict limitations.

SUMMARY

The most important fundamental errors of medicine are:
(1) Erroneous theories of aetiology. These are of two kinds: firstly, wrongly attributing symptoms to a hypothetical but non-existent pathological process or to an incidental pathological process or physiological variation and, secondly, making incorrect hypotheses about the cause of pathological processes.
(2) Assuming that treatment derived from theory must be effective - the supreme error of medicine. To a large extent this treatment was a consequence of erroneous theories of aetiology. Errors also resulted from theorizing about the effects of treatment.

In spite of all the controlled trials of treatment in recent years, many remedies of unproven value are still given for theoretical reasons, although those who advocate them may not state, or even be aware, that this is so.
(3) Forgetting the patient. When dealing with conditions clearly requiring surgery or with acute disasters the doctor can properly forget the patient and concentrate on the diseased part. Forgetting the patient leads to disaster when patients have long-standing and multiple symptoms.
(4) Over-valuing technology. Surgery, anaesthetics and much medical treatment are dependent on technology. And many valuable diagnostic measures need technology. But for the vast majority of patients technology is not relevant. Our error lies in over-applying it and over-emphasizing its importance. The other three errors are all traditional; this is the great modern error.

References

1. Stockman, R. (1920). *Rheumatism and Arthritis.* (Edinburgh: Green)
2. Asher, R.A.J. (1959). *Trans. Med. Soc. London,* **75,** 60
3. Leading article (1978). *Br. Med. J.,* **2,** 1736
4. Leading article (1979). *Br. Med. J.,* **1,** 505
5. Goyle, K.B. and Dormanby, J.A. (1976). *Lancet,* **1,** 1317
6. Cave, D.R., Mitchell, D.N. and Brooke, B.N. (1976) *Lancet,* **1,** 3111
7. Hilton, J. (1863). *Rest and Pain.* (London Bell & Daldy)
8. Beaumont, G.E. (1937). *Medicine. 3rd Edn.* (London: Churchill)
9. Percival, R. (1969). *Holland and Brew's Manual of Obstetrics 13th Edn.* (London: Churchill)
10. Lewis, T. (1942). *Diseases of the Heart. 3rd Edn.* (London: Macmillan)
11. Richardson, J.S. (Ed.) (1956). *The Practice of Medicine.* (London: Churchill)
12. Shulman, A., Shaw, F.H., Cass, N.M. and Whyte, H.M. (1955) *Br. Med. J.,* **1,** 1238
13. Leading article (1956). *Lancet,* **2,** 980
14. Cecil, R.L. (1943). *Textbook of Medicine.* (Philadelphia: Saunders)
15. Medical Research Council Committee (1948). *Br. Med. J.,* **2,** 769
16. Read, A.E. (1975) *Prescribers J.,* **15,** 91
17. Murray-Lyon, I.M. and Reynolds, K. (1976) *Br. Med. J.,* **2,** 923
18. St. John Sutton, M.G. and Rubenstein, D. (1974). *Br. J. Hosp. Med.,* **12,** 691
19. Matthews, D.D. (1977). *Br. J. Obstet. Gynaecol.,* **84,** 108
20. McMichael, J. (1979). *Br. Med. J.,* **1,** 173
21. Committee of Principal Investigators (1978). *Br. Heart J.,* **40,** 1069
22. Matthew, H. and Lawson, A.A.H. (1975). *Treatment of Common Acute Poisonings.* (Edinburgh: Churchill Livingstone)
23. Lawson, A.A.H. (1976). *Br. J. Hosp. Med.,* **16,** 333
24. Vale, J.A. (1978). *Prescribers J.,* **18,** 67
25. Todd, J.W. (1973). *Lancet,* **2,** 980

26. Todd, J.W. (1978). *Br. Med. J.*, **2**, 774
27. Matthew, H. (1968). *Prescribers J.*, **8**, 40
28. Leading article (1979). *Br. Med. J.*, **1**, 288
29. Leading article (1979). *Br. Med. J.*, **1**, 505
30. Asher, R.A.J. (1951). *Lancet*, **1**, 339
31. Pallis, C.A. and Bambi, A.N. (1979). *Br. Med. J.*, **1**, 973
32. Dornhurst, A.C. and Hunter, A. (1967). *Lancet*, **2**, 666

9

The Cults of Medicine

As the years go by the proportion of the GNP in the advanced countries devoted to health steadily increases. There is also an endless stream of books, articles and broadcasts about the advances of scientific medicine. Yet at the same time we are repeatedly told how deep is the dissatisfaction of the public with orthodox medicine, which is ineffective for so many maladies. We read about various kinds of fringe or alternative medicine, which are said to succeed when doctors fail. The President of the Faculty of Homeopathy of the Royal London Homeopathic Hospital stated[1] in a letter to the *British Medical Journal* (1979): 'As many doctors and patients are aware, there is at present a tremendous boom in the teaching and practice of all varieties of healing outside the conventional medical establishment. This has arisen from the mechanistic and specialized approach in much of modern medicine and the increasing concern of the public, and indeed of many doctors too, about the side effects, toxicity, and allergic reactions of many modern drugs.'

HOMEOPATHY

The most 'respectable' of the cults is homeopathy. Most of those who practise it are qualified doctors and for many years the British Royal Family has been treated by homeopathic physicians.

The originator of homeopathy was Samuel Hahnemann, who was born in Saxony in 1755. His great discovery was that 'likes should be treated by likes' or *similia similibus curentur*. Whereas orthodox doctors are *allopaths*, because they are said to believe in the opposite principle that a disease must be cured by an antidote.

After Hahnemann had qualified as a doctor in Leipzig he became, with every justification, dissatisfied with the bleedings, purgings, and other brutal remedies of the time. He practised in a swampy district, where the prevalent fever was known to respond to cinchona bark (from which quinine is obtained). According to Cullen's *materia medica,* which represented the orthodox view of the time, cinchona dealt with fever by its tonic effect on the stomach. Hahnemann did not agree with this view and took some cinchona bark himself, after which he developed the symptoms of the fever without the pyrexia. His family reacted in a similar way. A remedy that was effective for a disease thus induced symptoms of the disease in a healthy person. He then found that Hippocrates had said that substances which produced symptoms could also cure them.

After this Hahnemann spent many years in research to study the effects of various substances on the body, which he gave to his helpers and which he called the 'provings' of remedies. In this way he produced a *materia medica* from the vast number of his observations. An often quoted example of his provings is belladonna, which produced the symptoms and signs of scarlet fever. He therefore gave it to patients during an epidemic of this disease and the results were said to be spectacular.

Homeopathic physicians give their drugs in minute doses. One part of the drug is first mixed with 9 or 99 parts of an inert diluent, this being called the first potency, either 1X, if in the decimal scale, or 1C in the centesimal scale. The same manoeuvre is repeated, producing the second potency, 2X or 2C, and again repeated many times. Sometimes 'low' potencies such as 1X to 6X, and sometimes 'high' potencies, up to 200C or more, are used in practice. In the 'high' potencies the drug is so diluted that only one molecule may remain in several gallons of medicine. An explanation as to how a drug can have an effect in such incredibly minute amount was advanced[2] by Gibson: 'Emanations (of homeopathic potencies) have been demonstrated, and even photographed, electronically. The absorption of the 'dose' probably takes place directly from the mouth and may not be either by the blood stream or by the lymphatics but in some other way associated with nerve-force transmission'.

Another important tenet of homeopathy is that the patient as a whole, as well as his disease, should be studied. The homeopathic doctor also assesses the manner in which different patients react to the same infection. According to Margery Blackie[3] (1976), Physician to the Queen: 'In treating a patient with an acute chest infection no symptom is unimportant. If he lies on the affected side and is very thirsty, bryonia is indicated. Does he like someone near and needs to be reassured (phosphorus), or prefer to be left alone and resents disturbance (natrum sulph). Does he want all the doors and windows open, ignoring draughts (pulsatilla) or does he hate the slightest draught (hepar sulph). Is he frightfully cold and yet sweating profusely and wanting to be fanned (carbo veg). Is he exhausted by talking, very hot and putting his feet out of bed (sulphur). Does any patient feel worse at certain times of the day or night between 4 and 8 pm (lycopodium) between 2 and 4 am (kali carb). Whatever his complaints these are all very important points in finding the homeopathic remedy. One of our most important remedies is arnica. It is useful taken as a tablet every few minutes for any injury or bruising, mild or severe. It eases the pain very quickly. It is also useful after operation, in cases of undue exhaustion from travelling or for undue fatigue and lack of energy after certain heart conditions . . .'

Homeopaths make much of the undoubted fact that their medicines cannot do any harm. Whereas 'allopathic' medicines can do a great deal of harm from their side effects and sensitization reactions.

Is there any evidence that homeopathic remedies give any benefit over and above the placebo effect? In 1812 the survivors of Napoleon's army in its retreat from Moscow brought typhus fever with them. We are told that Hahnemann treated many of these men and achieved incredible cures, having only one fatality among 180 cases. In 1830 there was a cholera epidemic and whereas the orthodox physicians had a mortality rate of 55%, that of one of Hahnemann's pupils was only 4%. Modern homeopaths merely assert that their remedies 'cure'. Thus, Margery Blackie[3] (1976) states: 'for those of us who practise, it is known to be a safe and very effective treatment and often gives spectacular results'. Janet Watts[4] in the *Guardian* (1975) devoted an article to Dr Chandra Sharma, a leading homeopath. 'Dr Sharma was a highly qualified orthodox practitioner who knew of homeopathy only as a discredited quackery when he went to work at Great Ormond Street Hospital 30 years ago. He was suffering from a disease of the spinal cord that, he had been told, would paralyse him from the waist down in a year. Opposite his hospital was the Royal London Homeopathic Hospital. He was so impressed by its results with children that he moved there to work and also took homeopathic treatment for his disease. In six weeks it was cured. Dr Sharma now runs a successful London practice . . .'

All such anecdotes and assertions are of course totally valueless in assessing the value of a remedy. There is, indeed, no worthwhile evidence that any homeopathic remedy has any beneficial effect. There has been a complete absence of controlled trials. Margery Blackie[5] (1971) comments: 'We should welcome such (controlled) trials. Unfortunately, the nature of homeopathic treatment does not lend itself easily to that method of testing. The homeopathic approach is to treat the patient as a whole rather than the disease. So different patients may be treated by different medicines for a malady which non-homeopaths would generally regard and treat as the same in all of them'. But there would be no apparent difficulty in doing a satisfactory controlled trial of the management of, say, the common cold (which homeopaths say can be cured). All the patients would be seen by the homeopathic physician who would prescribe according to the personality and background of each one. Alternate patients would be given this prescription and the other would be given a placebo. If a trial could be arranged along these lines, and if there was unequivocal proof that the patients who were given the correct homeopathic remedy recovered from their colds more quickly than those who were given the placebo, the sceptics would indeed be forced to take homeopathy seriously. The onus of proof should rest upon the homeopaths, not upon the sceptics.

ACUPUNCTURE

The most ancient of the cults is acupuncture. There is documentary evidence of its continued use in China for 2500 years, though it is said to have originated thousands of years before that. According to Ilza Veith[6] (1972): 'All of Chinese medicine is based on the concept that, in composition and function, man is a microcosmic image of the universe and subject to identical universal laws'. The course of nature was thought to be guided by *Tao*, the Way, which 'causes the ever-recurring changes from day to night, from light to darkness, from life to death and is present in the co-existence of good and evil, of male and female. The two forces through which *Tao* acts were named *Yin* and *Yang*, with *Yin*, the female element, possessing all the negative and *Yang*, the male element, all the positive properties . . . In the universe, the harmonious working of the dual forces, *Yin* and *Yang*, expressed itself in the waning and waxing of the moon, the rising and setting of the sun, the growing and ripening of the crops and countless other sequential natural phenomena. Droughts, floods, storms, tidal waves, earthquakes and other disasters of nature were thought to be the result of an imbalance of *Yin* and *Yang*. Similarly, in man and beast, health resulted from the balance of *Yin* and *Yang*, and all diseases were thought to be an imbalance of these forces.

'In the physical body, both human and animal, the vital essence, *ch'i*, consisting of an appropriate mixture of *Yin* and *Yang*, was believed to be conveyed through 12 main ducts, described in the Western World as "meridians". The . . . meridians emerge to the surface of the body at a certain number (usually 365) of carefully designated and presumably sensitive places which subsequently became known as acupuncture points' .

'As a consequence of these beliefs, the Chinese did not recognize a variety of diseases. They saw only disease as such, brought about by one cause - the disequilibrium of *Yin* and *Yang* and the vital force - which could affect different organs and different parts of the body. Since the 12 meridians conveying the *Yin* and *Yang* were held to have a direct connection with every organ and part of the body, it was logical to assume that it was the meridians which furnished the easiest access to the seat of the disturbance. In response to the individual symptoms, specific points were chosen for each needling treatment. Each of the acupuncture points ... was directly related to a specific organ or portion of it. By inserting needles into one or several points and by leaving them *in situ* for a certain length of time, the equilibrium of *Yin* and *Yang* was expected to be restored, possibly by permitting the escape of disharmonious combinations'.

Whereas homeopathy and many other cults have been widely known in the Western World for many years, only during the last few decades have we heard much about acupuncture. Since then, there has been a spate of articles in the lay and medical press and broadcast programmes about the matter, and we are told of the great 'demand' for this treatment. *The Times* carried an article in 1962 by its medical correspondent[7] on 'Age-old conflict between *Yin* and *Yang*' and an article in 1974 by Dr Louis Moss[8] on 'Acupuncture: the medicine doctors seem determined to ignore'. According to Dr Moss 'many thousands of people who have been told that nothing further could be done for them and have been advised to live on aspirin and other pain killers have been greatly relieved of their pain and other disabilities'. Migraine, the chronic rheumatic diseases and 'the multitude of nervous disorders such as depression, nerve tension and insomnia' can all be relieved by acupuncture.

Felix Mann (1963) described the treatment of headache by acupuncture[9] and concluded: 'A series of 42 patients suffering from headache of various types, in which orthodox medicine had failed to effect much improvement, were treated by acupuncture. Of these, 32 were cured or showed considerable improvement, five patients showed moderate improvement, and in three there was no improvement or aggravation'. In his book *Acupuncture* (1962) Mann stated[10]: 'At any particular juncture, of all the 1000 or so acupuncture points possible to choose from, there are about 50 which, if stimulated with a needle, will help the patient (certain of these 50 more than others). On the contrary, there are about 50 which, if stimulated, will make the patient worse (certain of them even grievously ill), while the remaining 900 or so are more or less neutral'.

The most spectacular apparent success of acupuncture has been in producing anaesthesia. We have been shown on the TV screen Chinese people undergoing major surgery with no anaesthetic beyond acupuncture and they have lain passively still with no sign that they were feeling pain. This, to many people, supplies proof that acupuncture really does work. Perhaps all this fanciful talk of *Yin* and *Yang* is nonsense, it is said, but this doesn't alter the fact that it causes anaesthesia. But the important question is 'What is the "it" which is the responsible factor?'. Patients have had laparotomies under deep hypnosis. A possible explanation of acupuncture anaesthesia is that it is of similar nature to hypnosis. The matter could easily be put to test, without elaborate controlled trials, by trying to induce anaesthesia in exactly the same manner as usual by acupuncture, except that the needles are inserted in the wrong places. If it were consistently found that anaesthesia did not then occur, whereas it regularly occurred when the needles were inserted in the 'right' places, the sceptics would indeed be forced to admit that there is 'something in it'. Until this happens we can rightly believe that acupuncture anaesthesia is essentially the same as anaesthesia by hypnosis.

In assessing the value of acupuncture as a 'cure' for various maladies, we clearly need controlled trials. As well as comparing acupuncture with a placebo, we could again compare acupuncture with needles in the wrong places with it in the right places. Until these are done, we can rightly assume that acupuncture gives its benefits by suggestion.

OSTEOPATHY AND CHIROPRACTIC

Osteopathy and chiropractic are the most popular cults in the Western World, especially in the United States, where every small town has one or two practitioners.

Osteopathy began in 1874, when the American A.T. Still laid down the following principles: '(1) The body is self-sufficient to manufacture its own remedies, drugs being unnecessary. (2) The rule of the artery is absolute and universal and disease will result if it is obstructed. (3) All diseases are effects, the cause being a partial or complete failure of the nerves to conduct the fluids of life.' In practice, osteopaths are largely concerned with what are termed 'osteopathic lesions' in the spine. According to Stoddard[11] (1959): 'An osteopathic spinal lession is a condition of impaired mobility in an intervertebral joint ... the moment when irreversible pathological changes take place in the joint, it ceases to be a purely osteopathic lesion'. In the *Osteopathic Blue Book*[12] it is stated that: 'the lesion is not simply a bone malalignment, although in some cases this may well be the major evidence of its existence. Nor is it loss of movement alone, though some would attach great significance to this feature and deem it more important than positional abnormalities. From the layman's point of view, it could almost be described as a 'behaviour pattern' of a segment or section of the spine, involving the whole fabric of the skeletal structure'. It is also said in the *'Osteopathic Blue Book'* that 'the presence of spinal lesions exerts an influence upon the systems of the body through nerves and blood circulation ... and the existence of osteopathic lesions both predisposes a patient to disease and at the same time handicaps his natural powers of recovery'. These 'lesions' are held to be at least partially responsible for asthma, bronchitis, catarrh, sinusitis, peptic ulcers and constipation, and other alimentary disorders.

Chiropractic began on September 18, 1895 at Davenport, Iowa. On that day D.D. Palmer (an ex-grocer and fish peddler who for the previous 10 years had practised magnetic healing) was consulted by Harvey Lillard, who 17 years previously, when he exerted himself in a cramped position, had felt something give way in his back and at the same time became permanently deaf. Palmer found him to have a painful prominent vertebra and using the spinous process of the vertebra as a lever, applied a sharp thrust which 'repositioned' the bone. Shortly afterwards Lillard announced that his hearing had greatly improved. Thereafter Palmer abandoned magnetic healing and made his living by adjusting people's spines. He and his son established a College of Chiropractic at Davenport in 1895.

Chiropractic was defined, in a submission to the Massachusetts Legislature in 1966, as 'The science of locating and removing interference with the transmission or expression of nerve force in the human body, by the correction of misalignments or subluxations of the bony articulations and adjacent structures, more especially those of the vertebral column and pelvis for the purpose of restoring and maintaining health'. According to Dintenfass[13] (1966) the diseases amenable to chiropractic include arthritis, asthma, bronchitis, bursitis, colitis, the common cold, constipation, digestive disorders, dysmenorrhoea, hay fever, headache, hypertension, low back pain, mental illness, migraine and trigeminal neuralgia.

Whereas osteopaths refer to the osteopathic lesion and to manipulation, chiropractors speak of subluxations and adjustments. However, to the ordinary observer these appear to be merely semantic differences, the principles and claims of both cults being similar. On the other hand, Weiant[14] (1958) says: 'We hold no brief for osteopathy; it differs from chiropractic both in theory and practice and unlike chiropractic, it no longer claims to be a drugless profession'.

Most of the public who flock to osteopaths and chiropractors are probably unaware of the underlying principles of these cults and of the claims made to cure all manner of disease. The reason for their going is to obtain relief from pain, especially in the back, by being manipulated. Indeed, to a large extent manipulation and osteopathy (or chiropractic) have become identified. Many journalists, even those writing in the quality newspapers, use the words osteopathy and manipulation interchangeably. Katherine Whitehorn[15] in the *Observer* (1970) said: 'there is an association for osteopathy within the medical profession and plenty of ordinary doctors do a bit of manipulation on the side'. In *The Times*[16] (1971), under the headline, 'Osteopathy gains cautious acceptance by doctors' the medical reporter stated that 'The British Association of Manipulative Medicine has about 200 members, all of whom are doctors, who believe firmly in manipulations as a valuable treatment'. And according to Christine Doyle[17] in the *Observer* (1978): 'There arrives a day in many a backache sufferer's chronicle of "treatment" when his conventional doctor says, "You'll have to learn to live with it"'. Although some doctors, especially GPs, may recommend patients to the best known local manipulator, there are many who seem to imply that patients deserve what they get if they stray from the established medical wisdom'. Polly Toynbee in the *Guardian*[18] (1978) reviewed a recently published book by Brian Inglis, *The Book of the Back*. Among her statements were: 'Orthodox medicine has failed to provide any remedy'; 'Many doctors have been forced, reluctantly, to recognize that osteopaths somehow manage to do good', and 'They (the doctors) say that manipulation is dangerous'. Her article ends: 'Can the strength of opinion among humble patients desperately seeking a cure that works break the cartel of the monstrous regiment of doctors?'.

Doctors are, then, accused of objecting to manipulation on principle because it is outside the established orthodoxy. This is total nonsense. Never throughout my medical career have I met a single doctor who took this attitude. As a medical student in the thirties I was taught by a highly revered orthopaedic surgeon, A.S. Blundell Bankart, who regularly performed back and also foot, manipulation. And ever since then many orthopaedic surgeons and consultants in physical medicine have frequently manipulated backs. James Cyriax, who was consultant in physical medicine at St. Thomas' Hospital, has been a well-known advocate of manipulation for certain kinds of backache. His name, indeed, regularly appears when medical journalists are writing on backache, usually with the implication that he is a rare exception who has strayed from the paths of orthodoxy and is probably an osteopath at heart. Certainly, doctors deride the concept of the 'osteopathic lesion' and the other theories behind osteopathy and chiropractic. They also deride the claims that osteopaths and chiropractors can relieve or cure all manner of diseases.

Undoubtedly, backache is one of our commonest medical problems, being a major cause of absenteeism in industry among the middle-aged. There is a Back Pain Association in Britain which was largely responsible for the formation of a working group by the Department of Health. In *The Times*[19] (1978) it was reported that this group estimated that three million consultations with family doctors and one million visits to osteopaths and other practitioners are made each year in Britain on account of backache. It was also said that patients are 'dissatisfied' with back pain treatment. What, then, is the evidence that the 'cure' for backache is manipulation, as medical journalists habitually imply?

If every patient with backache could be given permanent relief by manipulation, there could be no argument about the matter. Everyone would be manipulated, and the back pain problem would disappear. The most that can possibly be said of manipulation is that it may give worthwhile relief to some patients with some kinds of backache. Is it, then, possible to define the kinds of backache for which manipulation will help, and the kinds of manipulation which are effective?

In Chapter 2, p. 29 I pointed out that an exact pathological diagnosis cannot be made in most cases of backache (though unfortunately in the past doctors have habitually made bogus diagnoses, such as fibrositis and sacro-iliac strain). It is impossible to be sure sometimes whether or not many patients have the most talked-of cause of backache, the 'slipped disc'. In many patients, especially those with long-standing pain, emotional factors play a large part. We also know that if no treatment is given, the vast majority of backache gets better in time. Here is a situation in which assessing the value of treatment is peculiarly difficult. When we are attempting to assess manipulation, there is the added problem that there is no question of having a double-blind trial. Finally, the act of manipulating has a considerable psychological effect on the patient, especially if he has faith in the treatment and the manipulator is a man of powerful personality.

There have nevertheless been various trials in an attempt to assess manipulation. Doran and Newell[20] (1975) analysed a multicentre trial in which 456 patients with low back pain were randomly allocated one of four treatments — manipulation, physiotherapy, corset, or analgesic tablets. Patients were assessed 3 months and 1 year after admission to the trial. There were no important differences among the four groups of patients in the duration and severity of their pain. A few apparently responded well and quickly to manipulation, but there was no way of identifying such patients in advance. One hears, indeed, stories of individuals incapacitated by back pain who have immediately and dramatically improved after manipulation, and in that situation a controlled trial is not needed to conclude that manipulation has been beneficial. But it is not possible to lay down criteria which determine for which patients manipulation is especially indicated.

Osteopaths and chiropractors claim that they have a special expertise in manipulation or adjustment. In the *Osteopathic Blue Book* it is stated that: 'Proper skill in manipulation can be acquired only by years of diligent practice based upon systematic training. The student must acquire, among other things, a sense of precision, timing, localization and tension, together with an aptitude for measuring force, weight, angulation, stress and flexibility with accuracy'. Statements of this kind are not susceptible to proof. And the mind boggles at the thought of trying to devise an experiment to determine whether manipulation by an 'expert' is better than that by a beginner, when the condition being treated is infinitely variable in severity, is usually undiagnosable, and the main or only criterion of assessment is pain.

Difficult though it is to reach a firm conclusion about this matter, manipulation of the back appears to be beneficial sometimes. And perhaps doctors should manipulate more than they do. But this has nothing to do with the truth or otherwise either of the principles behind osteopathy or chiropractic or of the expertise of those who practise these cults.

NATUROPATHY AND HERBALISM

Even today, when we have so many successful 'cures', people recover from the vast majority of maladies by the natural processes of healing alone. And when there is an effective remedy, nature still plays an essential part in the healing process. When someone has a lacerated wound, the surgeon excises damaged tissue and sutures the skin edges together, which makes it possible for the patient to be left with a neat scar. But the actual healing of the wound is done by nature. When someone has lobar pneumonia penicillin may save his life, but he still needs his white blood corpuscles and other bodily defences.

Some of our present-day maladies can rightly be attributed to 'unnatural' ways of living. In the distant past there were few obese people yet today obesity is one of the commonest problems. It is due to a combination of under-exercising and over-eating, both of which can reasonably be called unnatural behaviour. Under-exercising also contributes to many other maladies, notably coronary artery disease. As to what constitutes an 'unnatural' diet will be further considered below, but one feature which can be considered unnatural, the removal of fibre from cereals, plays a part in diverticular disease and appendicitis and probably of piles and varicose veins. Whether or not smoke is unnatural is debateable and the houses of our primitive ancestors were full of smoke, whereas ours are not. But the belching of smoke by chimneys in cities, causing smogs, seems most unnatural and is responsible for much ill health. However, in this respect we are now living more naturally than we were 30 years ago. Tobacco smoking can also be called unnatural. A common cause of ill health has been alleged to be the 'stress and strain' of modern life. That too may be thought unnatural, though one can express grave doubts as to whether we pampered moderns suffer more stress and strain than did our primitive ancestors. We often read of 'stress diseases', though the evidence behind this theory is meagre. Another important cause of ill health is alcohol. When drunk in moderation alcohol can be considered natural, but excessive drinking can reasonably be described as unnatural.

In the light of all this the attractions of the nature cult are evident. If we would only live more naturally our state of health would be far better. And on most occasions when we are ill we would be just as well off, and sometimes much better off, if we had no treatment but just waited until nature made us well.

But naturopaths do not just tell people to do what they like and eat what they like (provided they don't get fat), take no drugs and leave the rest to nature; if this were all they did no-one would consult them. On the contrary, they advocate all sorts of remedies which they claim are nature's way of healing.

An idea which pervades naturopathic writings is that the body becomes clogged with accumulated 'filth' from years of unnatural living. Thus, Harry Benjamin[21] (1936) states: 'The first and *most* fundamental principle of nature cure is that *all forms of disease* are due to the *same cause,* namely the accumulation in the system of waste materials and bodily refuse, which has been steadily piling up in the body of the individual concerned through years of wrong habits of living, the chief of these being wrong feeding, improper care of the body, and habits tending to set up enervation and nervous exhaustion, such as worry, overwork, excesses, and abuses of all kinds'.

The means by which 'filth' is eliminated from the body are fasting and dieting, colonic lavage, deep breathing and other exercises, massage and various kinds of physiotherapy and perhaps 'natural' herbal remedies'. Homeopathic remedies may also be thought 'natural' and osteopathy to be a 'natural' form of treatment. Rich people go to extremely expensive nature cure establishments where these methods of treatment are carried out. One of the most famous of these in Britain was at Champneys (a former Rothschild mansion) near Tring, run by Stanley Lief. The cure usually begins with near fasting, and later 'natural unspoilt food', such as raw vegetables and fruits, are eaten.

Naturopathy, homeopathy, and osteopathy are, indeed, very much interlinked. There is a British Naturopathic and Osteopathic Association. In *Woman's Own*[22] (1976), under the heading, 'Just look what natural healing can do . . .', we are given an account of the triumphs of Dr Chandra Sharma, 'one of the world's leading homeopaths who once treated the Queen', in curing a 22-year-old top model with hypothyroidism. (Dr Sharma is also mentioned above, p. 174). Dr Sharma agreed with the orthodox doctors that the model was hypothyroid, but he explained that this was caused by delayed shock after the break up of her marriage, the hormones being unable to deal with the crisis. 'You must start with a fast', he told the model, so for a few days she had no food, but just sipped water. Then Dr Sharma worked out diets for her, 'altering them to suit each change in chemical balance . . . For 3 days I ate a handful of grapes, then I'd take 2 pounds of potatoes a day without salt or butter. After that a diet of yoghourt and orange for breakfast, green vegetables for lunch, and steak for dinner'. After a year she was pronounced cured and thereafter needed no thyroxin, though a few months before the year was up she went through a 'healing crisis', at which point Dr Sharma used acupuncture needles on her spine. 'The next day my period started, I hadn't had one for over a year, so at that moment I knew I'd get well'.

No doubt many of those who take the cure in one of the Nature Cure resorts are benefited. During the time they are there they do not as they probably do at home, overeat and in consequence they shed some excess fat. They take exercise, which they avoid in their everyday lives, and they cease from smoking. And their psychological state may well improve when they are away from their usual worries. But whether or not they derive permanent benefit is another matter. Most probably return to their old habits of eating too much, smoking and taking no exercise, and soon regain the weight they had lost.

A popular aspect of the nature cult is that food should be grown by nature's methods, that is, the proper fertilizers of the soil are compost and animal dung, no 'chemicals' of any kind being used. Views of this kind appear to be increasing and they are much more widespread than is the belief that ailments should be cured by nature's methods. There are increasing numbers of health food shops, where the eggs are free range and the vegetables are organically grown. Much ill health is attributed to the use of chemicals in farming. Organically grown crops are believed to be more 'nutritious', whatever that means, than those grown with chemical fertilizers. The same belief is held about free range eggs and chickens by comparison with the battery varieties. And all additives such as colouring agents and preservatives are condemned.

There is of course a modicum of truth in these beliefs. Many sprays are highly poisonous. Some insecticides kill bees and other useful insects. DDT, which was widely used as an insecticide some years ago, had ill effects throughout the animal kingdom. Nitrogenous fertilizers are leached into rivers, where they encourage the growth of undesirable plant life, which may choke everything else. Some food additives have been found harmful, or possibly harmful, to man and have been withdrawn. But nothing could be more absurd than the blanket condemnation of chemicals in general because one chemical in particular is, or may be, harmful. Each compound should be separately assessed on its merits.

The blanket condemnation of refined foods is equally absurd. Some kinds of refining, notably the removal of fibre from cereals, have been shown to have ill effects, but this supplies no proof that other kinds of refining are harmful. There is here the important practical problem that many people insist on eating white bread; to them wholemeal bread may be thought nasty, unclean stuff fit only for animals. Yet to many people, myself included, wholemeal bread is far superior in flavour to white bread. I have regularly eaten it since childhood, long before the benefits of bran were publicized, because it tastes so much better.

There is constant confusion in the public mind between the appearance and flavour of food and its 'nutritive' qualities. No doubt the flesh of battery chickens is often tasteless, but there is absolutely no evidence that this affects its 'nutritive' qualities in any way. And statements that 'natural' food tastes better are suspect. One reads repeatedly that free range eggs taste better than battery eggs. This could easily be put to test by asking a large number of people to say which poached egg is battery and which free-range when given one of each. Until such a test is done I shall continue to believe that the two kinds of eggs are indistinguishable by their flavour.

The belief in the superior qualities of the 'natural' product is indeed widespread. Many people buy Still Malvern water in bottles at considerable expense, which they regularly drink in preference to the cheap product out of the tap (which has been treated by all sorts of chemicals). Still Malvern is advertised as the 'purest water known'. But it is much less pure, and more expensive, than distilled water. Not only, therefore, is the addition of 'chemicals' bad; the artificial absence of chemicals in distilled water is also inferior to their natural absence in Still Malvern water!

In so far as the followers of the nature cult use remedies, these are, if not homeopathic, derived from herbs. In the not so remote past all doctors largely prescribed herbs, or simple tinctures and extracts derived from herbs. There remains a deep belief in the healing qualities of herbs. And there are still many herbalists throughout the affluent world.

We were informed by Robert Eagle[23] in the *Observer Magazine* (1978) that John Hyde, public relations man for the National Institute of Medical Herbalists, claims: 'Herbs will cure anything. And they don't have side effects', though he later qualified this by declining to say that he had a cure for cancer. He stated that there are only 50 herbal practitioners (as distinct from ordinary herbalists) who, being members of the National Institute of Medical Herbalists, 'can be trusted to prescribe herbal remedies responsibly'. We are told that about 200 plants are regularly used in herbal medicine in Britain.

Like homeopaths, acupuncturists, and osteopaths, herbalists claim that they treat people rather than diseases. A remedy prescribed at John Hyde's Herbal Clinic in Leicester contains up to 30 herbal tinctures, some of which would be aimed at symptomatic relief and others at the whole system. 'Antibiotic literally means anti-life', says Mr Hyde. 'We would treat many infections with *Rumex crispus*, yellow dock, which increases the white blood cells rather than attacking particular organisms. In this way resistance lasts long after the infection has passed'. The preparation of herbal remedies is said to make critical differences to their activity. 'Fresh comfrey root, for instance, is full of edible fibre and thus a good laxative, but marinated and made into a tincture it is used as a cure for diarrhoea.'

Herbalists maintain that in prescribing the pure compound which has been isolated from a herb, which is the standard practice in orthodox medicine, many of the natural benefits are thrown away. We are told that rauwolfia or snakeroot has been used for centuries in India as a sedative and a means of reducing blood pressure. A few decades ago an active alkaloid of rauwolfia, reserpine, was isolated and for a time was widely used by doctors in treating people with hypertension. And it was proved that the drug did lower the blood pressure. Unfortunately, it was liable to cause depression and its use was therefore largely abandoned. Herbalists say that the natural rauwolfia contains a vast assortment of compounds, in addition to reserpine and that, acting together, they are more effective than reserpine, without causing depression.

Like other kinds of fringe medicine herbal remedies are unlikely to do harm. But, whereas we can be certain that a homeopathic preparation cannot do harm, there can be no such certainty about herbal remedies. Nature provides poisons as well as 'cures'. We have all heard of deadly nightshade and the toadstool *Amanita phalloides*.

Evidence from controlled trials which demonstrates the value of herbal remedies does not exist. But there would be no difficulty in arranging satisfactory double-blind trials. Whole rauwolfia could be compared with reserpine by making 2 identical looking bottles of medicine, one containing reserpine alone and one containing rauwolfia in which there is the same amount of reserpine. If patients taking the mixture were less liable to depression and other side effects, while having a similar drop in blood pressure, this would be clear evidence that the mixture is superior to reserpine alone. Herbalists have complained that official bodies, such as the Medical Research Council, are uninterested in their remedies. But if they would carry out a trial and this clearly proved that a complicated mixture is superior to a single compound, the medical world would be forced to take notice.

HEALING

The essence of healing is treatment by spiritual means. The healer usually lays his hands on the sick person and by prayer, the relaying of some 'vital force', or some kind of 'spirit control' he is healed. On the other hand, it is also said to be possible to heal patients who are far away by the power of thought. A few gifted individuals are said to discover in themselves that they possess the power to heal. Thus, we are told[23] by Robert Eagle (1978) that Gilbert Anderson, the Secretary General of the World Federation of Healing, discovered his healing faculty by accident 30 years previously. 'I had a lot of trouble from a spinal injury during the war', says Mr Anderson, 'and had resigned myself to spending the rest of my days in a wheelchair. My wife persuaded me to go to a healer, and, much to my surprise, he cured me. Not long afterwards I was travelling round the country and by some chance, wherever I went I came into contact with desperately ill people. Within half an hour of my seeing them they made remarkable recoveries. At first I thought it was coincidental, until it happened every day for several weeks'.

One of the most famous of all healers was Harry Edwards. Geoffrey Moorhouse gave an account[24] of his powers in the *Guardian* (1966), describing him as 'the most celebrated spiritualist healer in Britain' who 'believes that he is a medium for the spiritual ministrations of Louis Pasteur and Lord Lister'. He used to see about 50 patients a week and also had about 1000 requests for healing *in absentia;* 'these he deals with in the small hours of the morning when, he says, he can be quiet and concentrated'. 'He reckons to obtain satisfactory results in 80% of all the cases he tackles and to produce a complete cure in 30% of those successful attempts. He has, he believes, cured people of practically any ailment or disease you care to name, including cancer. When he cures them in person he merely runs his hand over the sickened part of the body or manipulates a limb. When he cures *in absentia* he simply concentrates his mind on them; sometimes he is conscious of heat passing through his fingers to the patient's body; as often as not he is aware of no particular sensation at all.'

Geoffrey Moorhouse comments that there are even more astonishing claims than those made by Harry Edwards. Thus, 'A week or two ago the 'Psychic News' reported from the Philippines how a spiritualist healer removed a malignant tumour from a man's stomach without the benefit of surgery. According to this report he made a cutting movement with his fingers to open up the patient's abdomen; he severed the intestines with a pair of scissors but rejoined them manually; then his hand 'swished' over the incision and the skin closed again without leaving a scar'.

For many years members of the National Federation of Spiritual Healers have been allowed into many NHS hospitals, provided they were invited by the patient and did not interfere with the medical treatment. I should certainly not have objected to such a healer seeing one of my patients. But throughout my consultant career I had no single request, either from a patient or a relative, for the services of a healer. Robert Eagle[23] informs us that 'A few doctors, most of them GPs, are now working with members of the National Federation of Spiritual Healers in an attempt to find whether healing has any measurable benefit for cancer patients. One of these doctors, who was given 6 months to live after refusing to undergo radiotherapy after a cancer operation, went to a healer instead and is now alive, well and cancer-free, five years later'.

Healing is very much the concern of the Churches and is often thought to be inseparable from religious faith. The then Archbishop of Canterbury, William Temple, set up a committee in 1944 to examine spiritual healing. And an Archbishop's Commission in 1958 approved the development of the Anglican Church's ministry of healing. By far the biggest exercise in healing through religious faith takes place at Lourdes. Thousand upon thousand of sick people make pilgrimages there and the main means of livelihood of the townspeople is to house and feed them. Yet many healers deny that religious faith is a necessary part of healing. Harry Edwards took this attitude, and damned the manifestations which take place at Lourdes.

If a patient has profound faith in a healer, whether or not in a religious context, without doubt his symptoms can be greatly relieved by the healer's activities. When the patient is a victim of migraine or of various kinds of backache, he may apparently be 'cured'. Even if he has advanced multiple sclerosis, widespread cancer, or other unpleasant bodily disease, he may derive profound relief of his symptoms.

But the important practical question is: 'Is there evidence that

the actual course of organic disease can be changed by a Healer?'.
Can we accept that Harry Edwards could 'cure people of practically
any ailment or disease you care to name, including cancer?'. Here,
full and detailed information about patients is needed and they must
be observed over a long period. Such evidence is lacking. It is true
that isolated instances can be found of patients who were
undoubtedly affected by advanced cancer and apparently
recovered. A famous example was John Eagan, who had been
found to have advanced abdominal cancer at operation in Glasgow
in the 1960s, proved histologically. Prayers were said for him in
Catholic churches, urging the Blessed John Ogilvie (who had been
martyred in the early 17th century) to intercede on his behalf. He
made a complete recovery, and remained well for years thereafter.
John Ogilvie was later canonized.

The occasional isolated case of this kind is indeed remarkable.
But cases are also seen who have apparently recovered from
advanced disease without seeing a healer or having any other
treatment. I was concerned with such a case a few years ago. A man
was referred to me with numerous enlarged lymph glands and the
blood picture of acute leukaemia. To be on the safe side, I repeated
the blood count and it was unchanged. The patient was over 70 and
an advanced chronic bronchitic and I advised that the kindest
course would be to leave well alone. 3 months later I inquired from
the man's GP when he had died, to be told that he had not died but
was far better. I therefore saw him again and all his lymph glands
had gone and his blood picture was normal. Thereafter, there was
never any evidence of leukaemia. However, some 3 years later he
developed a swollen tonsil from which a biopsy was taken, showing
the appearances of lymphosarcoma. He was given radiotherapy
followed by striking shrinking of the lump but some months later he
died. Had he been seen by a healer when he showed the picture of
acute leukaemia, he would have seemed a spectacular example of
the healer's powers.

PSYCHO-ANALYSIS

Whereas the cults previously considered appeal to all strata of the population, psycho-analysis is the cult of the intelligentsia, especially in America. Freud first used the term psycho-analysis in 1896 and every educated person 'knows' that he was one of the great figures of history. Like Galileo, Copernicus, Newton and Darwin, he is said to have caused a revolutionary change in our ideas. We speak of the pre-Freudian and post-Freudian epochs. Terms coined by Freud, his disciples, or his rivals, such as *oedipus complex*, *inferiority complex*, the *unconscious mind*, *introvert*, and *extravert*, have become part of the language of the educated classes.

Perhaps the supreme Freudian concept is that of the unconscious mind. Deep inside our minds activity is said to go on of which we are never aware, or of which we can occasionally obtain fleeting glimpses by our slips of the tongue or our dreams. But by the help of a trained analyst we may in time be helped to obtain some insight into what is happening in our unconscious.

What kind of evidence is there, then, for the existence of the unconscious mind? A universal experience is to be unable to remember the name of a person or object with which one is familiar. If, after thinking hard without success for a time the matter is dismissed and the mind engaged otherwise, when an hour or two or a day later one again considers the problem the missing name is immediately recalled. This one simple observation seems to provide proof that some kind of activity can occur in our minds without our being aware of it. In the psycho-analytic world mental activity at this level is defined as preconscious. But there is also the 'true unconscious', which consists, says Ernest Jones[25] (1948), of 'thoughts which are quite incapable of becoming conscious unless a special manipulative activity is brought about by an analytic procedure'.

'Proof' of the reality of the 'true unconscious' can, then, only be produced by the activities of an analyst. How can it be proved that the interpretations made by the analyst are correct? To do this there must be some kind of evidence entirely independent of analysis. Such evidence does not exist and until it is produced the question as to whether there is a 'true unconscious' cannot be answered.

Analysts maintain that the study of dreams provides some of the evidence for the existence of the 'true unconscious'. According to Freud, the manifest dream is derived from latent dream thoughts by a mechanism which he called the dream-work. And he maintains that the function of all dreams is to preserve sleep and that their formation 'may be either a wish-fulfilment, or its opposite, an anxiety or a punishment, brought to actuality' (1929)[26]. Hypotheses of this kind are unprovable.

Freud lays down the symbolic interpretation of various objects and activities which occur in dreams. Thus, many objects symbolize the male genitalia, or the penis alone, including sticks, trees, pointed weapons of all kinds, the figure 3, firearms, taps, watering cans and certain reptiles and fishes, notably the serpent. Dreams of flying are erection dreams. Pits, caves, jars, boxes, chests, pockets, rooms, doors, snails, the mouth, and churches symbolize the female genitalia. Pubic hair symbols are woods and bushes. Piano playing, sliding, gliding, and pulling off a branch are symbols for masturbation. Blossoms and flowers are symbols for virginity. Sexual intercourse is symbolized by dreams of being run over and such rhythmic activities as dancing and riding. Apples, peaches, and other fruits symbolise the breasts. Emperors, empresses, kings and queens are the dream symbols for parents. Clothes and uniforms symbolize the opposite state of nakedness. And so on.

One of the most celebrated of Freud's beliefs was the importance which he attached to childhood sexuality. A kind of sexual activity is said to begin in babyhood with an *oral phase* of sucking and swallowing. Towards the end of the first year the oral phase is overlapped and succeeded by the *anal phase*. There is then strong interest in the excreta, this being the period when the ability to control the anal sphincter develops. At the end of the third year this pregenital sexuality gives way to the genital or *phallic phase*.

During the phallic phase the male child's interest is centred on his penis and is associated with feelings of sexual attraction to his mother and jealousy towards his father - the famous *oedipus complex*. Alternatively, there may be an inverted oedipus complex, when the boy is attracted to his father and jealous of his mother. 'There is no possible doubt', says Freud, 'that one of the most important sources of the sense of guilt which so often torments neurotic people is to be found in the oedipus complex'. And, says Ernest Jones[25], 'All other conclusions of psycho-analytic theory are grouped around this complex and by the truth of this finding psycho-analysis stands or falls'. The oedipus complex fades out about the fifth year, chiefly because the boy fears that his desire for his mother may be punished by his father with castration (which here implies the loss of the penis rather than of the testes). This is the *castration complex,* which will, says Freud[26], 'play such a large part in the formation of his character if he remains healthy and of his neurosis if he falls ill'.

In girls the oral and anal phases are said to be similar to those in boys. During the girl's phallic phase she becomes interested in her clitoris, but since this is obviously inferior to the masculine organ develops the desire to be a boy. This is the phase of *penis envy,* which in psycho-analytic circles is thought most important. Later, the girl becomes reconciled to castration and renounces the life of masculinity. She may now develop the *electra complex,* with attachment to her father and jealousy of her mother, though this is given much less emphasis than the oedipus complex.

When a new baby arrives in the family his brothers and sisters are said to be deeply jealous of him. He may have to be kept away from them, since otherwise they might do him actual physical harm. This is *sibling rivalry.*

The difficulties experienced by a child in passing through the pregenital phase of development are believed, in psycho-analytical theory, to have a fundamental influence on his character. Fixation at or regression to one of these phases are thought to be responsible for neurosis. Thus, says Otto Fenichel[27] (1945), 'Psychoanalysis of stutterers reveals the anal-sadistic universe of wishes as the bases of the symptoms. For them, the function of speech regularly has an anal-sadistic significance. Speaking means, first, the utterance of obscene, especially anal, words and, second, an aggressive act directed against the listener ... As in the case of tic, the anal orientation in asthma is also closely related to tendencies rooted in still earlier phases of development. Asthmatic patients turn out to be passively-receptively directed, orally and temperature - erotically dependent, possessed by a very great narcissistic need to regain their lost omnipotence'.

A distressing mental malady of children is autism. This has similarities with schizophrenia and the child is withdrawn, lacks emotion, and seems unaware of the outside world and may repeat meaningless phrases. In psycho-analytic theory it is due to the 'rejection' of the child by the mother who subconsciously wishes that he did not exist. In recent years it has been brought home to all how widespread is parental cruelty to children. There are endless cases of 'child abuse', in which children are burnt, thrown around the room, starved and subjected to other horrific cruelties. Yet such children as these do not become autistic. The mother of the autistic child may be intelligent and apparently looks after him with tender, loving care. Yet, we are told, she is actually 'rejecting' him subconsciously and he is so aware of this that he retreats into his own private world of phantasy.

Whatever are the attractions of psycho-analytic theory to some, or its absurdity to others, from the patient's standpoint the important practical question is: 'Is it effective in practice?'. There are no controlled trials to help us and the advocates of psycho-analysis can only supply anecdotes about individuals to support their claims. Such anecdotes are worthless as a means of assessment. To make the situation more difficult, whereas when dealing with the diseases of the body there may be objective phenomena, such as the presence of a lump or the level of the temperature, to help us to make an assessment, when dealing with the disorders of the mind we must almost entirely depend on the symptoms. In this situation it can be very difficult even to decide whether or not a patient has improved; to decide whether improvement has been due to treatment is impossible. In any case, the psychological state varies widely according to the circumstances of the individual or for no apparent reason, whether or not he is having treatment.

The only way in which we can gain any idea as to whether psycho-analysis is likely to be beneficial is, then, to look at what happens in the analyst's consulting room. A full analysis involves some three or four interviews per week for perhaps 3 or 4, or even 7 or more years. At each interview the patient usually lies on a couch in a quiet room, the analyst sitting outside his range of vision. The analyst encourages him to reveal all his innermost thoughts, without selection or suppression. Many of these thoughts are likely to be painful and involved with intense disturbing emotions. The analyst therefore tries to help him to overcome his 'resistance' to these disturbing emotions. Analysts state that in the short run the release of such emotions may actually worsen the patient's state. During the analysis, the patient may develop a powerful emotional relationship with the analyst. He may feel alternatively love and hatred or dependence or rejection. This relationship (which is thought to reflect the patient's relationships with his parents, siblings, and peers of childhood) is called the transference. Usually it is said to be positive at first, reflecting the patient's gratitude towards the analyst. Later, or sometimes throughout the analysis, the transference may be negative, the patient's feelings being intensely hostile, this hostility (provided it is not permanent) being thought a valuable release mechanism. The handling of this transference situation is believed to reflect the expertise of the analyst.

Melanie Klein, one of the most famous analysts, has described[28] in her book, *Narrative of Child Analysis* (1961), a detailed account of the analysis of Richard, a 10-year-old. The following are typical extracts.

'R. feared there might be a collision between the sun and the earth and the sun might burn up the earth; . . . the earth . . . was so important and precious . . . He . . . commented how awful it was what Hitler did to the world . . .'

'Mrs K. interpreted that the "precious earth" was mummy, the living people her children . . . the sun and earth in collision stood for something happening between his parents. "Far away" meant nearby, in the parents' bedroom . . .'

'R. expressed his fears about the British battleships being blockaded in the Mediterranean . . . He wondered how the British troops could be rescued from Greece.'

'Mrs K. interpreted that he also worried unconsciously about what might happen to Daddy when he put his genital into Mummy. Daddy might not be able to get out of Mother's inside and would be caught there, like the ships in the Mediterranean. . . .She referred to what he had said in the first session about a person standing on his head and dying because his blood flowed down. This is what he thought might happen to Daddy when at night he put his genital into Mummy. He was also afraid that Mummy would be hurt by the tramp - Daddy. Thus he felt anxious about both parents and guilty because of his aggressive wishes against them. His dog Bobby stood for himself wanting to take his father's place with Mummy (the armchair standing for the bed) and whenever he felt jealous and angry, he hated and attacked Daddy in his thoughts. This made him also feel sorry and guilty (oedipus situation) . . .'

'R. looked at the map upside-down and commented what a "funny" shape Europe had when looked at that way. He said it was "not proper" and seemed muddled and mixed up'.

'Mrs K. linked this with parents, "muddled and mixed up" in sexual intercourse so that he could not make out who was who when he thought of them in this situation. She also interpreted his fear that in sexual intercourse the parents became so mixed up that the bad Hitler-penis inside Mother remained in her (combined parent figure). This was what he meant by "not proper", "funny" and he actually felt it to be bad and dangerous. . . . .'

'R. showed anxiety. He . . . looked around the room . . . He picked up Mrs K's clock.

'Mrs K. interpreted that this exploring the room stood for the wish to explore her inside, due to his anxiety to find out whether there was a Hitler-penis in it or a good one. Therefore he asked about Mr K. All this linked with Mummy and with the mixed up parents . . . .'

'R. was very pleased to see Mrs K. . . .on the way . . .he twisted his ankle. He asked Mrs K. to look at his new suit. Didn't the colour of his socks go well with it?

'Mrs K. interpreted that his twisting his ankle . . . was an expression of his fear that he would injure his genital if he fulfilled his desire to be a man and put his genital into Mrs K's genital. When he pointed out his new suit to her and asked her to admire his socks, he also shewed the wish for her to admire his genital. But that was followed by his fear that he was no good at all . . . that he would never have the adult and effective genital that he wanted . . .'

'R. drew battleship *Nelson,* submarine *Salmon* . . .starfishes, babies.'

'Mrs K. interpreted that the portholes (on *Nelson*) also represented babies, as did the starfishes . . . He wanted Mummy to have many babies . . . when they tore out the bad octopus, this meant that he and Paul were tearing father's bad genital out of Mummy, and that he and Paul tore the Hitler-penis out of Mrs K. The salmon which made Mummy ill over the weekend was also Daddy's bad genital. The port-holes meant having easier access to Mummy's body . . . The plant to which the babies wanted to be near stood for Mummy's breast, her genital, and her inside . . .'

'The fear of the internalized dangerous penis is a strong incentive for testing out this fear in external reality and strengthening homosexual desires. If anxiety with the internalized dangerous penis is very strong, such reassurance is of course not obtained, and this may lead to an obsessional increase in homosexuality . . .'

'I have made much in my *Psycho-analysis of Children* of the combined parent figure which, I suggested, plays a vital part in the early stages of the oedipus complex (between 4 and 6 months). I concluded . . . that if this combined parent figure is strongly maintained in the infant's mind, this influences both the sexuality and the whole development of the child. One of these phantastic figures is the mother containing the penis of the father, or many of his penises. Further observations suggested that there are even phantasies in the very young child about the mother's breast containing the father's penis and this phantasy usually contributes to a disturbance of the love for the breast and to a diminished belief in its goodness . . .'

'R. said that the mind was even more important than the body, though he thought the nose was very important too'.

'Mrs K. interpreted that the nose also stood for R's genital and that he was afraid that something was wrong with it, that it was damaged and would not develop properly and this was the reason why he was afraid of becoming a "dunce". He doubted whether Mrs K. could actually cure the genital as well as the mind.'

What possible comment can be made on this passage?

Especially in the United States, only a very rich elite can afford psycho-analysis. According to Gross[29] (1978) some 30 000 people in the United States and perhaps another 10 000 in the rest of the world are undergoing analysis - among the millions of the mentally disordered. No doubt many of those who have spent vast numbers of dollars over the years to be analysed in the end believe they have benefited. They may be satisfied that the 'insight' they have acquired about their symptoms has given them a fuller understanding of their own natures. They may accept, for example, that their oedipus complex has persisted or that they have a powerful castration complex. No doubt Richard, the boy analysed by Melanie Klein, and his parents realized that when he looked around the room he was really wanting to explore Mrs K.s inside to find out whether there was a Hitler-penis or a good penis in it and that when he twisted his ankle he was expressing a fear that he would injure his genital if he fulfilled his desire to be a man and put his genital into Mrs K's genital. But all this proves is that the analyst has persuaded the patient to accept certain beliefs; it does not prove that the beliefs are true.

OTHER CULTS

In addition to the cults already discussed, there are many lesser-known ones in the Western World, and more of such cults in the East.

Mathias Alexander introduced the Alexander Principle to Britain in 1904. Among his followers were Lily Langtry, Bernard Shaw, and Stafford Cripps. The aim of the Principle is to correct the damage we do to our bodies by tensing muscles. Wilfred Barlow of the Alexander Institute[30] says: 'consider that 85% of the population have arthritis in the neck by the time they are 50 and half the adult population get severe back pain. It comes from bad use of the body and muscle tension and my aim is to teach people to forget bad habits, not to teach new exercises . . . the body balances from the head. If that is thrown out everything else is distorted'. The patient, or pupil, as he is called, attends courses which teach him a new style of muscular use known as 'body grammar'.

Shiatsu is a 700-year-old Japanese method of massage and physiotherapy. Its main purpose is to correct faulty circulation and activate organs that have ceased to function properly. This is achieved by finger and thumb pressure on 'vital nerve endings'. Success is claimed in treating asthma, stomach ulcers, arthritis, migraine, sinusitis, and insomnia.

Aromatherapy is, we were informed by Derek Malcolm[31] in the *Guardian* (1967), 'a back and head massage, based on German spinal massage and Chinese acupuncture and assisted by the introduction through the skin of oils which help recuperation from run-down conditions and are claimed to possess remarkable curative powers'. Madame Marguerite Maury is a leading exponent of aromatherapy. Tracy Clair[32] in the *Guardian* (1966) reports Madame Maury as saying that she found 'a veritable treasure trove of information in Hindu, Chinese and Tibetan sciences'. Every patient is said to need a different blend of oils 'to help her retain the glow of youth'. 'To arrive at the individual prescription Mme Maury photographs different areas of skin and enlarges them; she takes blood samples for crystallization and examination. So far, she is the only person able to make these diagnoses'.

'Nerve manipulation' was a method of treatment used by Ernest Stephan between the Wars. Jean Soward[33] in the *Sunday Express* (1967) informs us that this treatment had been revived by Peter Stephan, the son of Ernest. 'The technique is based on the ancient Indian art of removing tension and so wiping away anxiety lines, scowl marks and other signs of the passing of the years, through a special kind of massage of the deep nerve centres.' 'I apply various degrees of pressure to the nerve centres around the spine', says Mr Stephan, 'and the result is a noticeable and *automatic* relaxation of the patient'.

A Bio-Energy Centre, we were informed by Vicki Mackenzie[34] in the *Observer* (1978), was set up by Gerda Boyesen, a Norwegian physiotherapist and psychoanalyst, in 1968. Peg Nunneley, who learned her massage technique from Gerda Boyesen, claims that 'there is an energy field which exists throughout all the living world...This is the energy used in acupuncture, the energy referred to in Yoga, the energy which has been photographed by the Kirlians in Russia'. This energy 'gets blocked when it meets tensions' but when Peg Nunnerley has heard through her stethoscope the changes in the body's energy balance she is 'guided to place her hands where the tension is'. And by her massage she enables the energy to flow again. Migraine, rheumatoid arthritis, diabetes, hay fever, sinusitis and constipation are among the maladies successfully treated.

Culliton and Waterfall (1979) report[35] that the Laetrile movement has accelerated astonishingly in the United States since 1970. Laetrile is an apricot derivative which, it has been estimated, has been taken by 75 000 Americans in the belief that it will cure cancer. Evidence that it gives benefit is totally lacking.

In 1945 there was one Thalassotherapy Institute in France; by 1967 the number had grown to 15, most able to deal with 300 or more clients daily. Jean Soward[36] (1967), in the *Sunday Express* says the principle of the sea beauty cure is that 'Fresh deep sea water contains the same mineral elements as the fluid under the skin in which our body cells live and are nourished. Plunge the body into cold sea water and the pores close ... Heat this same water, however, to several degrees above natural body temperature and the pores dilate. The skin now acts like a sponge, drinking in the mineral-filled sea water giving a sort of "cocktail" fillip to our often depleted fluid. Our cells receive the elements they lacked and start to function vigorously again'. This, combined with massage from a hot sea water jet and a 'healthy' diet, is said to be a natural rejuvenator.

An important aim of many cults is, indeed, to make people young again. From time immemorial men have sought, and some have claimed to have discovered, the Elixir of Youth. The ancient Egyptians were said to ward off old age by making themselves vomit and sweating profusely. In Roman times the breath of young maidens was thought to have the same effect. In the 18th century the Count of St. Germain claimed that by drinking his 'Tea of Long Life' people could achieve an age of 2000 years. In my childhood a man who regularly filled the newspapers was Dr Serge Voronoff who used 'monkey glands' to rejuvenate old men. These 'glands' were chimpanzee's testicles, which he grafted into his patients. Although this had no effect, thereby he achieved fame and fortune.

A current Elixir of Youth is cellular therapy. Sylvia Matheson[37] (1966), in the *Times,* described the work of the Zurich physician Dr Franklin E. Bircher, who had treated, among others, Charlie Chaplin, Gloria Swanson and Conrad Adenauer. Dr Bircher's method was to 'regenerate' diseased and failing organs by the injection of a 'series of live hormone cells taken from freshly killed, specially bred sheep'. He initially does 'rigorous tests', some devised by himself, 'of every bodily organ'. After collating the results he 'selects the sheep from the healthy, tested flock under his personal supervision and removes the living cells himself, which must be used within one or two hours at most'. These injections are repeated according to the individual's 'needs' and finally 'massive doses of vitamins' are injected into the blood stream. Within weeks or a few months 'the body responds to the effects of the injections, the eyes sparkle, the hair becomes more lustrous and vital, the complexion clears and the net result is a generally younger appearance ...' Sylvia Matheson, who had the treatment herself, 'no longer suffers from rheumatism' and her 'general health has been absolutely first-class'.

The originator of 'cellular therapy' was Professor Paul Niehans, who was even more famous than Dr Bircher. He is said to have treated the Duke and Duchess of Windsor, Somerset Maugham, the Japanese Imperial family, Marilyn Monroe, Pope Pius XII and General De Gaulle. Neil Lyall and Robert Chapman (1976) in the *Sunday Express* tell us[38] that his practice was 'to determine the type of cells in which a patient appears to be deficient, and inject a solution of appropriate or matching sheep cells to boost areas in need of them. The injected cells reach their target by a sort of natural 'magnetic attraction'.

In 1959 Prof. Ana Aslan of Romania became briefly famous in Britain because of the rejuvenating effect of GH3 (usually known as procaine). She had treated various high dignitaries in the communist world. And, according to Lyall and Chapman, Dr Hewlett Johnson, the Red Dean of Canterbury, visited her clinic in Bucharest when he was over 80. He said: 'I had a course of her treatment which had an extraordinarily happy effect on me, restoring powers that I had lost. It made me feel and act as if several years had been taken off my age'. Clinical trials of GH3 were carried out in Britain and it was found to be totally ineffective.

Radionics is, we are told[23] by Robert Eagle (1978), 'a form of distant healing which relies on as yet unexplained paraphysical energies. The practitioner usually never sees the patients, let alone examines them. Diagnosis is performed by swinging a pendulum over a lock of hair or spot of blood and treatment is effected by beaming out paraphysical energy with the help of an instrument made from magnets and variable resistors'. Radionics was discovered by Dr Albert Abrams of San Francisco, who died in 1924.

Finally, various individuals have their own particular 'cures'. Barbara Cartland[39] (1973) says: 'An enormous number of people stop being sexy very early in life because they're not eating the right things. White sugar is the curse of civilization - it causes fatigue and sexual apathy between husband and wife. My recipe against sexual fatigue is to take honey in large quantities, two Gev-E-Tabs, ten vitamin E pills, four wheatgerm oil tablets, four vitamin A pills, four bonemeal tablets, six liver-plus tablets and two dessertspoons of Bio-Strath Elixir, twice a day'. And, we are told by Ena Kendall[40] (1975) in the *Observer Magazine* that Mrs Julia Owen treats people by stinging them with bees 'fed with special medicaments based on the fungi produced by dried egg and milk fermented in whisky, wine and different herbal saps and mixed with honey according to the individual needs of patients'. She is mainly successful in restoring the sight of those blind with retinitis pigmentosa, but she also cures 'arthritic and rheumatic diseases, ... weeping eczema, dermatitis, ... asthma, hay fever, sinusitis and diabetes in patients who have not had insulin'. Mrs Owen 'gave up hope of recognition from the medical profession long ago'. 'Tell them to go to hell', she said.

THE APPEAL OF THE CULT

In Chapter 8 I advanced the view that two of the great errors of medicine over the ages were to devise bogus theories of aetiology and to base treatment on theory, either a theory of aetiology or a theory about the effect of the treatment. And because so much treatment has done so much harm, the second error is the supreme one. But in recent years we have made these errors much less often than in the past. Bogus theories of aetiology have mostly died and it is widely accepted that the only sound test of a remedy is the empirical test of whether it is effective in practice.

All these cults are based on one or both of these errors. Homeopathy depends on the principle of treatment *similia similibus curentur*. Acupuncture depends on the theory of aetiology that illness is due to an imbalance of *Yin* and *Yang* and on the theory of treatment that by inserting needles in the right places this imbalance can be rectified. Osteopathy depends on the theory that an 'osteopathic lesion' in the spine is responsible for all or many illnesses, and that by manipulation of the spine health can be restored. Naturopathy depends on the theory that disease is due to unnatural habits of living and that its cure is achieved by remedies, including herbs, which are deemed natural. Healing depends on the theory that by spiritual means organic disease can be made to disappear. Psycho-analysis depends on the theories that our unconscious minds profoundly influence our behaviour, that we all pass through specified phases in our sexual development, and that neurosis is due to disorders of this development. And by the help of an analyst, who can give us insight into our unconscious, our neuroses can be cured. The other cults are dependent on similar theories.

Untold thousands of people are convinced that they have been 'cured' or relieved by the remedies given by those who practise these cults, which explains their popularity. Throughout the ages the public were equally convinced that the medical profession cured their maladies, but nearly all the treatments prescribed by doctors more than 50 years ago are extinct. We know that, so far from being beneficial, many were harmful and the remainder were useless. Patients recovered not because of, but in spite of, the doctor's remedies. The mere observation, therefore, that people are convinced of the value of the cults in itself proves nothing.

The appeal of psycho-analysis for the intelligentsia has long been an especial puzzle to me. Eminent professors, distinguished authors and learned historians do not believe that the earth is flat or that we are regularly visited by spacemen from other worlds. Nor do they believe in astrology, poltergeists, fairies, witches, ghosts or even the long-range weather forecast. Yet they may swallow, hook, line, and sinker, the astonishing doctrines of Freud and his followers, for which there is no better evidence than there is for these other beliefs. Thus, they accept that we all as children pass through the oral, anal and phallic phases in our developing sexuality, that all boys are affected by the oedipus complex and girls feel 'penis envy', and that in our dreams many objects symbolize the male genitalia and others the female genitalia and that dreams have a 'purpose'. They also accept the remarkable interpretations of ideas and behaviour, such as those of Melanie Klein in the analysis of the boy Richard (as recounted above, p. 195). Psycho-historians, instead of spending long years in studying ancient documents or digging in archeological sites, as do their foolish brethren, can write their biographies without leaving their desks, just by the exercise of imagination. Freud himself set the trend[41] in his 'Leonardo da Vinci'. Here he made all sorts of astonishing deductions from the following single early memory of Leonardo: 'It seems that I was always destined to be so deeply concerned with vultures; for I recall one of my very earliest memories that while I was in my cradle, a vulture came down to me and opened my mouth with its tail and struck me many times with its tail against my lips'. (In fact,

Leonardo's memory was of kites, not vultures, an error arising from a mistranslation of the original Italian into German).

Perhaps, in the words of Arthur Koestler[42] in his autobiography (1952), the attraction of Freudianism is that, like Marxism and Catholicism, it is a 'closed system'. 'By a closed system', says Koestler, 'I mean, firstly a universal method of thought which claims to explain all phenomena under the sun and to have a cure for all that ails man. It is, further, a system that refuses to be modified by newly observed facts but has sufficiently elastic defences to neutralize their impact, that is to make them fit the required pattern by a highly developed technique of casuistry. It is, thirdly, a system which, once you have stepped inside its magic circle, deprives your critical faculties of any ground to stand on. The last point is perhaps the most important. Within the closed system of Freudian thought you cannot, for instance, argue that . . . . you doubt the existence of the so-called castration complex. The immediate answer will be that your arguments are rationalizations of an unconscious resistance which betrays that you yourself have such a complex. You are caught in a vicious circle from which there is no logical escape. Similarly, if you are a Marxist and if you claim that Lenin's order to march on Warsaw in 1920 was a mistake, it will be explained to you that you ought not to trust your own judgement because it is distorted by vestiges of your former petit-bourgeois class-consciousness. In short, the closed system excludes the possibility of objective argument by two related proceedings: (a) facts are deprived of their value as evidence by scholastic processing and (b) objections are invalidated by shifting the argument to the psychological motive behind the objection. This procedure is legitimate according to the closed system's rules of the game which, however absurd they seem to the observer, have a great coherence and inner consistency'.

Underlying this discussion is the implication that assessing the value of treatment can be a matter of extreme difficulty. People recover from the vast majority of maladies with the aid of nature alone. Any treatment is given the credit which nature deserves. Symptoms, and especially pain, are relieved by the placebo effect of treatment. If the patient is sufficiently convinced that someone, whether doctor or not, has especial skill he will on that account alone be benefited. And if the giver of the treatment has a powerful personality and is convinced that he himself can cure people, this effect will be all the greater. Yet when some remedy is overwhelmingly successful, it is easy to know this, without elaborate double blind controlled trials. If the malady is a chronic unvarying condition, such as hernia or prolapse, which disappears after an operation, we know for certain that the operation was successful. And we know that cyanocobalamin cures pernicious anaemia, that penicillin cures syphilis, and that PAS, streptomycin and isoniazid cure tuberculosis.

The difficulties of assessment arise when dealing with recurrent and variable conditions when there is no consistently effective remedy. And people with conditions such as migraine, dyspepsia, asthma, backache, 'rheumatism', neuroses etc. provide most of the clientele of the practitioners of cults. But if everyone with backache could be permanently cured by manipulation, every victim would be manipulated and the back pain problem would have been solved for ever.

We habitually read in the lay press and even at times in the medical press that modern doctors are less cocksure than they used to be (which we must hope is true) and that therefore they look more kindly on 'alternative' or 'fringe' medicine than they did. In the *Guardian* (1978) appeared this headline: 'Fringe medicine is beginning to break through the barriers of medical scepticism'. In the ensuing article Vicki Mackenzie[43] made the following statements. 'Fringe medicine is . . . being tentatively accepted into the very fortress of conventional healing - the National Health Service'. 'Acupuncture is now being used in a big London Hospital to relieve patients of pain'. 'One leading physician . . . prefers to remain anonymous until he has consolidated his experiments with bioenergetic massage for the relief of hypertension'. 'David Ennals . . . has met a group of Natural Therapists to hear how unorthodox medicine could promote health'. 'For 15 years (a 60-year-old consultant physician) has prescribed . . . flower and herbal potions. "I give (he says) mustard to help depression, pine for guilt feelings, star of Bethlehem is good for shock and primulus for fear . . . What they do, unlike drugs, is treat the basic problem itself, not just the symptom". He also practises acupuncture . . . it seems to work particularly well in relieving asthma and migraine . . . At the moment he is studying homeopathy too . . . "I do believe it is possible to direct energy mentally", he says'. '(Acupuncture) seems particularly effective (says a consultant anaesthetist) on diseases like arthritis, low back pain and migraine'.

On the other hand, we sometimes hear it suggested that doctors will get into trouble if they stray from the paths of orthodoxy. They will, perhaps, be hauled before the BMA and told that if they don't behave themselves they may lose the right to practise. We also read that doctors as a body are most conservative. Werner Pelz[44], in the *Guardian* (1966), says: 'Long ago and far away ... there lived an unqualified medical practitioner. One day ... he cured a man of his blindness by means of a concoction not mentioned then or since in acceptable textbooks. His patient was duly hauled over the coals by the Medical Association of the day, known to us only under the cover-name of "Pharisees". The patient could but repeat, "What he is I do not know. But while I was blind, now I can see". For such stubbornness he was debarred from all future welfare benefits, for then as now, the orthodoxy of Medical Associations puts to shame all other orthodoxies. Adamantly, it affirms *semper et in saecula saeculorum,* that he who has not been cured by the approved method cannot have been cured'.

Among all the attacks that are made on the medical profession, perhaps the most absurd is that we are all orthodox and conservative, that we all accept the same doctrines. This may have been true in past centuries when to deviate from Galen was forbidden, but present-day doctors vary infinitely in their views and change them repeatedly. By contrast, the unalterably orthodox are the fringe practitioners. A homeopath must believe that *similia similibus curentur;* otherwise he will have to abandon all his cherished beliefs. And an osteopath who ceases to believe in the osteopathic lesion is no longer an osteopath. Anyone who regularly gives the same treatment, even if it is valuable sometimes, inevitably gives it too much. That is why I advanced the view (see Chapter 7, p. 120) that the specialty of radiotherapy is unsatisfactory, because it is a specialty of treatment.

Medical journalists repeatedly write about the side effects of the treatment prescribed by doctors. There are numerous articles about the side effects of the Pill alone. The public has been so often told about the occasional disastrous brain damage attributed, probably in many cases wrongly, to whooping cough vaccine that the proportion of children vaccinated against all the childhood infections has markedly dropped. Whereas we are constantly told that the practitioners of alternative medicine do no harm. This is of course largely true. Many drugs do have serious side effects and doctors prescribe vastly too many drugs. A drug given in such dilution that only one molecule remains in several gallons, which happens in homeopathic prescribing, cannot possibly do harm. One cannot be so sure about herbal remedies, but probably nearly all are harmless. Laying on of hands and other forms of healing are totally benign. It has been alleged that people have acquired hepatitis from acupuncture needles, but this can only happen if they are not sterilized between patients; otherwise acupuncture is harmless (apart from the brief pain it causes). If, therefore, someone has a malady for which no treatment should be given - and this is true of most maladies - he will do better by going to a fringe practitioner who gives him a nonsensical but harmless treatment than by going to a doctor who wrongly gives him a prescription.

Another repeated complaint made by medical journalists against doctors is that they never have time to listen; they just shut the patient up by handing out a prescription. No doubt this is all too often true and is a grave reflection on the medical profession. Whereas the fringe practitioners are said to be more sympathetic and to be willing to listen. The repeated claim is also made by the fringe practitioners that they treat the patient, not just the symptom. This is largely meaningless verbiage. If a patient has one symptom which can be completely and permanently abolished, there can be no better treatment than to abolish it. Medical students are brought up with the doctrine that a most awful mistake is just to treat the symptoms. They may be regaled with tales of appalling GPs who have given patients chalk and opium for their diarrhoea instead of inserting a finger into the rectum and discovering a carcinoma. Of course, many doctors, specialists in particular, do spend too much time in concentrating on the system from which symptoms arise and too little time in sitting back and looking at the patient as a whole (as I have emphasized throughout this book).

THE INFINITE GULLIBILITY OF
MEDICAL JOURNALISTS

A prime function of the press is to expose scandals. If medical journalists can find things wrong with the medical profession they are doing a public duty by airing them. And they have no difficulty in finding things wrong since doctors themselves habitually attack each other. In this book I have been harshly critical of my own profession. We read endlessly about iatrogenic illness, of which a large number of hospital in-patients are said to be suffering. Any doctor who claims that the treatment given by his colleagues is wrong can be sure of getting press publicity. Medical journalists as a body are, indeed, highly critical — and sometimes rightly critical — of the medical profession.

But when medical journalists are writing about alternative medicine, they take a very different line. They regularly accept without question the wildest claims that people have been 'cured' of all kinds of diseases by the machinations of some practitioner of alternative medicine.

If an editor were sent articles which showed how to turn base metals into gold or which demonstrated a perpetual motion machine we can be reasonably sure that he would turn them down. But when sent articles claiming to have discovered that other great dream of the mediaeval alchemist - the Elixir of Youth - he may publish them without qualification. This is true, not just of the popular press, but of the most distinguished journals. As noted above (p. 200) we were informed [37] in the *Times* that Dr Bircher regenerates diseased and failing organs by injecting 'live hormone cells' taken from freshly killed sheep, carefully selected by himself. Similarly, in the *Guardian*, Elisabeth Dunn (1972) described the work[45] of Peter Stephan (who in 1967 was giving 'nerve manipulation', see above, p. 199) who gives injections of animal cells at £200 per treatment which are said to be 'The Secret of Eternal Youth'. Indeed, the *Guardian* habitually gives free puffs to 'cures' which one might have thought would have looked suspect to the most callow journalist. Marguerite Maury (see above, p. 199) the aromatherapist[32] is 'the only person able to make these diagnoses' (through studying skin photographs and blood samples) by which individuals can be prescribed a particular blend of oils which help her 'retain the glow of youth'. In 1973 we were informed by Janet Watts[46] in the *Guardian* that Mrs Betty Roney can cure, or at least arrest, baldness by 'diet, massage, exercise, massage (sic), homeopathy, medical and herbal remedies, nature cure, vitamins, and infra-red lamps, as the individual case requires'. In this way she 'beats the quacks at their own game'. And in the *Observer*[34] (see above, p. 199) we were told of Peg Nunneley, who can hear through a stethoscope 'the changes in the body's energy balance' and thereby gives massage to enable the energy to flow again.

SUMMARY

(1) Many of the public, dissatisfied with orthodox medicine, go to those who practise 'fringe' or 'alternative' cults.

(2) The main cults are homeopathy, the most 'respectable', acupuncture, the most ancient, osteopathy and chiropractic, the most popular, naturopathy and herbalism, healing or treatment by spiritual means and psycho-analysis, the cult of the intelligentsia. There are also innumerable minor cults, notably those which claim to have discovered the Elixir of Youth.

(3) All cults are based on one or both of two great errors of medicine: devising bogus theories of aetiology and devising treatment from theory - either a theory of aetiology or a theory about the effect of treatment.

(4) People often believe that they have been 'cured' by the treatment given by cult practitioners for the same reason that they used to believe that they were 'cured' by the useless of harmful remedies of doctors in the past - patients recover from most maladies by nature alone. When people are treated by someone of strong personality whom they believe to have special skill they may on these accounts be benefited.

(5) Assessing the value of treatment is most difficult when dealing with such recurrent and variable conditions as migraine, dyspepsia, asthma and backache. Patients with such conditions especially go to cult practitioners.

(6) Doctors have widely varying views; the views of cult practitioners are unalterable.

(7) People affected by maladies not helped by treatment may do better by consulting a cult practitioner (who gives them a harmless remedy) than by seeing a doctor (who wrongly prescribes a potentially harmful drug).

(8) Medical journalists are often rightly critical of doctors but are infinitely gullible when writing about cults.

References

1. Boyd, H.W. (1979). *Br. Med. J.*, **1**, 821
2. Gibson, D.M. *Elements of Homeopathy.* (London: British Homeopathic Association)
3. Blackie, M.G. (1976). *Times*, September 1
4. Watts, J. (1975). *Guardian*, April 17
5. Blackie, M.G. (1971). *Br. Med. J.*, **2**, 586
6. Veith, I. (1972). *Modern Medicine*, 12 November
7. Medical correspondent (1962). *Times*, June 16
8. Moss, L. (1974). *Times*, August 30
9. Mann, F. (1963). *Med. World*, **98**, 284
10. Mann, F. (1962). *Acupuncture. The Ancient Chinese Art of Healing.* (London: Heinemann)
11. Stoddard, A.S. (1959). *Manual of Osteopathic Technique.* (London: Hutchinson)
12. *Osteopathic Blue Book.* London.
13. Dintenfass, J.D. (1966). *Chiropractic. A Modern Way to Health.* (New York: Pyramid Books)
14. Weiant, C.W. (1958). *Medicine and Chiropractic.* (New York: Augustin)
15. Whitehorn, K. (1970). *Observer*, November 8
16. Medical reporter (1971). *Times*, December 8
17. Doyle, C. (1978). *Observer*, July 23
18. Toynbee, P. (1978). *Guardian*, July 17
19. News item (1978). *Times*, May 15
20. Doran, D.M.L. and Newell, D.J. (1975). *Br. Med. J.*, **1**, 161
21. Benjamin, H. (1936). *Everybody's Guide to Nature Cure.* (London: Health for All)
22. *Woman's Own* (1976). July 20
23. Eagle, R. (1978). *Observer Magazine*, May 21

24. Moorhouse, G. (1966). *Guardian,* March 5
25. Jones, E. (1948). *What is Psycho-analysis?* (London: Allen & Unwin)
26. Freud, S. (1929). *Introductory Lectures in Psycho-analysis.* (London: Allen & Unwin)
27. Fenichel, O. (1945). *The Psycho-analytic Theory of Neurosis.* (New York: Norton)
28. Klein, M. (1961). *Narrative of Child Analysis.* (London: Hogarth)
29. Gross, M.L. (1978). *The Psychological Society.* (New York: Random House)
30. Barlow, W. (1973). *Alexander Principle.* (London: Gollanz)
31. Malcolm, D. (1967). *Guardian,* July 13
32. Clair, T. (1966). *Guardian,* December 12
33. Soward, J. (1967). *Sunday Express,* April 9
34. Mackenzie, V. (1978). *Observer,* January 8
35. Culliton, B.J. and Waterfall, W.K. (1979). *Br. Med. J.,* 1, 802
36. Soward, J. (1967). *Sunday Express,* August 13
37. Matheson, S. (1966). *Times,* May 31
38. Lyall, N. and Chapman, R. (1976). *Sunday Express,* September 19
39. Cartland, B. (1973). *T.V. Times,* April
40. Kendall, E. (1975). *Observer Magazine,* February 16
41. Freud, S. (1975). *Standard Edition of the Complete Psychological Works.* (London: Hogarth)
42. Koestler, A. (1952). *Arrow in the Blue.* (London: Hutchinson)
43. Mackenzie, V. (1978). *Guardian,* June 23
44. Pelz, W. (1966). *Guardian,* October 13
45. Dunn, E. (1972). *Guardian,* April 7
46. Watts, J. (1973). *Guardian,* December 21

10

The Future of Medicine

Attempts to prophesy what will happen in future invite ridicule, since no-one can anticipate the discoveries that are going to be made. Nevertheless, it is useful to hypothesize developments which could happen in the light of present knowledge. We can also extrapolate present trends, since these can be expected to give a reasonably accurate guide to the near future and some guide to the more distant future.

As I noted in Chapter 4, in the affluent societies we have both the power and the knowledge to improve our state of health very greatly. We all know that if we never smoke, drink only in moderation and do not drink and drive, restrain eating to the extent that we never become obese, and take plenty of vigorous exercise, we will live several years longer and enjoy better health. We also know how we can avoid venereal disease and how we can make road, work and home accidents both less likely and less damaging.

In Chapter 5 I pointed out that doctors have it in their power to make a vast reduction in the cost of the curative health services. GPs could reduce their prescriptions to a fifth or less of the present figure with nothing but benefit. GPs could also be more restrained in ordering investigations and in referring patients to hospital, and in particular they could decline to give way automatically to every 'demand' of patients to see a specialist. Thereby the pressure on hospitals would be greatly eased.

Hospital doctors could reduce the number of investigations done to a fraction of the present figure, and cease altogether from doing 'routine' investigations. They could only send to the Intensive Treatment Unit those few patients who benefit from being there, and they could greatly diminish the amount of very expensive but so often inappropriate treatment, such as intravenous feeding and blood transfusion. They could much reduce the number of prescriptions. Physicians could stop the admission of walking patients for investigation and retain those admitted as emergencies for a shorter time. And they could much reduce the number of 'old' out-patients. Surgeons could be more restrained in advising operations of doubtful value and do far more outpatient surgery and keep many patients in hospital for much shorter periods. Radiotherapists could confine their attentions to that fairly small number of patients who are likely to derive more good than harm from radiotherapy and cancer-chemotherapy.

On the other hand, if we extrapolate present trends, the future looks dismal in the extreme. The public are drinking more alcohol as the years go by and more and more road accidents are drink-related. Obesity is probably still increasing. Some of the health-conscious middle class appear to be exercising more, but overall the amount of exercise taken is probably declining. The incidence of venereal disease, other than syphilis, is going up. The only favourable trends — and these are slight — are in tobacco consumption and diet. There has been a small drop in smoking and an increase in the amount of roughage, especially bran, eaten. We may hope these trends will continue at an accelerating rate.

The medical picture is even more dismal. GPs overall are not prescribing less and are referring as many or more patients to hospital. Investigations are still increasing. More and more advanced technology is used in investigations, notably in the nuclear field and in computer-assisted tomography. The proportion of the GNP devoted to the curative services continues to increase.

Are there any prospects of a reversal in these trends? One possibly hopeful sign is the suggestion recently of some disenchantment with High Technology. Perhaps doctors will become more critical both of investigation and treatment than they have been in the past. If they fail to do so, financial restraints may increasingly force attitudes to change (as to a slight extent they have already done). If pathology and X-ray departments are set strict cash limits they will be compelled to find ways of lessening the number of investigations. Clinicians in turn will have to stop ordering enormous numbers of tests without a thought as to the cost. Such financial restraints are bound to be unpopular. If they are used, one can envisage high medical dignitaries solemnly warning the politicians that patients' lives are being put at risk.

Perhaps the simplest and most effective way of making the best use of short-term hospital beds would be to appoint in all hospitals medical superintendents who are empowered to lay down policies on bed use. This system was used in municipal hospitals in the pre-NHS days, and, provided the medical superintendent was tactful and always discussed changes of policy with his colleagues, was said to work well. Over the years I have often discussed this matter with colleagues and many have thought that there would be much to be said for having a medical superintendent to make day to day decisions instead of the present system, or lack of it, when no-one seems to have clearly defined responsibilities and trivial problems are shunted from committee to committee. It must nevertheless be feared that some consultants would revolt if attempts were made to reintroduce the office of medical superintendent.

THE INCREASING MECHANIZATION OF MEDICINE

Whatever happens in future, there is bound to be further mechanization and computerization. A prophecy of what the future may be like is given in the following passage from 'Medical Judgement - the Master Computer' by Seabord[1] (1968).

'For several days you have not been feeling well and you call your local health centre for an appointment. You can remember when you used to call your doctor, but it's been many years since he's bothered with initial diagnoses and he would be the first to admit he could not be as thorough or accurate as the health centre. At the centre you give all the necessary information to a medical secretary whose typewriter feeds it into a computer system ... On the basis of the information given so far and a comparison with your previous history the computer may venture an immediate diagnosis, but if it has any doubts - and it is a highly conservative computer - it recommends one or several diagnostic tests ... In a matter of seconds ... the system presents its full diagnosis. At the same time it also makes recommendation for treatment, perhaps printing out a prescription which can be filled before you leave the centre. Fortunately, in your case only medication was recommended and you go home not only with the proper medication but confident that your case was given the best medical attention, even though you never saw a doctor during the entire visit. The health centre efficiently adds the day's information to your medical history and sends your doctor a copy just for the record. By the way, you do get to see your doctor - on the weekend when you play bridge with him.'

Of course, much technology has been a genuine advance and has benefited patients. The supreme modern medical error has been the over-valuation of technology and its inappropriate use (see Chapter 8, p. 163). In only a minute proportion of occasions when a patient seeks medical help is high technology needed; in practice it may be applied as routine.

Implicit in the accounts or prophecies as to how computers could take over from doctors is the fallacy of the single word or phrase diagnosis and the specific treatment. In practice the single phrase diagnosis is sufficient with some acute illnesses such as 'malaria' or 'perforated peptic ulcer' and in these examples the treatment too is fairly clear-cut. And when patients have malignant disease the single phrase diagnosis is of overriding importance, though the decision as to treatment may involve all kinds of subtle considerations. But when patients have many minor acute maladies and all long-standing benign maladies the single phrase diagnosis becomes absurd. Patients with persistent or recurrent backache, bellyache, or headache, general malaise, exhaustion, palpitation etc. can only be diagnosed, if at all, in a sentence. And the question of specific treatment hardly arises. In Chapter 7, I have advanced the view that on the vast majority of occasions when someone seeks medical advice the best person to deal with the situation is the general practitioner, who looks at the patient as a whole against his background. Whatever discoveries are made in the future and whatever advanced machines are developed, this will always remain true. One of the main benefits we can hope of new discoveries is that they will better enable the GP to select the few patients who should be investigated or referred from the many patients who should not.

Although the idea that doctors will be replaced by sophisticated machines which make diagnoses and prescribe the correct treatment is absurd, more and more elaborate machines which replace various organs or parts of the body will continue to be produced. The most strikingly successful machine so far is the dialyser which replaces the failing kidney. The latest home models enable people to live reasonably normal lives at the expense of being attached to the machine with arterial and venous cannulae for a few hours two or three times per week. No doubt continued improvements will be made in these kidney machines.

A contributory explanation of the success of the kidney machine is that kidneys need not function continually. Other organs to which this applies are the liver and gut. Is there any possibility that machines which take over the function of the liver and to which the patient is attached at intervals, will be evolved? Although the difficulties are immensely greater than in the case of the kidney, it seems conceivable that success may ultimately be achieved. We already have means of replacing the gut - by intravenous feeding of the essential elements. There is unlikely to be much improvement in this field.

But even the best of all machines outside the body is intrinsically unsatisfactory. What we need is a machine inside the body which replaces failing organs. Is it conceivable that we can ever have an internal artificial heart, lung, kidney, liver, or endocrine gland? The problems to be solved are so immense that any success must be in the remote future. Perhaps the most attractive possibility is the artificial heart, since the function of the heart is so much simpler than that of the lung, kidney, liver, or gut. We already have heart machines to which the patient is temporarily attached while cardiac repair is carried out. Ultimately technology may possibly enable us to operate electric pumps inside the body.

The parts of the body that are already replaced by inanimate substances include teeth and joints. And the total hip replacement can be brilliantly successful in giving complete relief of pain and improved mobility to the victims of osteo-arthropathy. Continuous efforts are being made to provide similar knee, elbow, ankle, wrist and finger joints. No doubt some success will be achieved. But replacing living tissue by the best tolerated of all inanimate substances always gives rise to problems.

Kidney-grafting has been one of the most spectacular developments of recent years. And this has great and obvious advantages over intermittent dialysis. Are there any prospects that the intrinsic difficulty of grafting — the rejection of the graft by the recipient — will ever be overcome completely? Immense amounts of research have already been carried out in this field, with only very limited success. Cylosporin A is a new substance which gives promise of achieving a marked improvement. As we are here dealing with a fundamental property of animal life, it seems very doubtful if the rejection problem will ever be totally solved, though prophecy in so complex a field is unwise.

In Britain one important reason why many unfortunate patients who are suitable for kidney grafting are not given grafts is the shortage of cadaver kidneys. The problem is difficult. The biggest source of kidneys is young people who die in hospital shortly after being involved in road accidents. There are all sorts of reasons why their kidneys are not in practice used. Those who work in hospitals are unwilling to interview relatives who are in extreme distress and to request permission to remove kidneys from their loved ones. The situation would no doubt be improved if the law were so altered that it would become legal to remove organs from the dead unless instructions objecting to this were left by the dying person. But there would be strong opposition to such a change in the law, if for no other reason than the near-impossibility of ascertaining whether in fact the dead person had left instructions.

Without reasonable doubt the future will also see an increase in the number and improvement in the results of grafting other organs, including the liver, lungs, and heart. Heart-grafting has had enormous publicity but is currently rarely being attempted except by Shumway and his team in California. But whereas kidney grafting has already made a worthwhile impact, these other grafts have not. Liver grafting may well become a useful procedure in future. But I venture to prophesy that lung and especially heart grafting are never likely to provide a practicable means for treating more than a tiny proportion of the victims of pulmonary or cardiac failure.

POSSIBLE NEW CURES

Although it is idle to speculate about new cures which are at present undreamed of, it is reasonable to consider which maladies are potentially curable and which are not. We can be sure that we shall never be able to cure various kinds of advanced disease. If someone has had a stroke, leaving him aphasic and hemiplegic, we shall never be able to bring his dead brain back to life. And if someone's joints are destroyed by rheumatoid arthritis, we shall never be able to make them normal again. We can be almost as pessimistic about the prospects of curing disseminated malignant disease. However, even today we can sometimes successfully ameliorate widespread prostatic and mammary cancer by hormone therapy. And acute leukaemia, which is one type of disseminated malignant disease, can sometimes be 'cured'. It is therefore conceivable, if unlikely, that drugs will be discovered which eradicate disseminated carcinoma without doing irreparable harm to other tissues.

The most striking triumph of curative medicine in the recent past has been the anti-bacterial drugs. Few people in the affluent world now die from bacterial infections, leaving aside the terminal infections of the elderly. The most obvious prophecy about the future is that we will develop drugs which cure viral illnesses. And although many viral illnesses are minor, such drugs would bring great benefit. It would be best of all if we could prevent the common cold. But failing this, a drug taken as soon as the cold began which promptly aborted it would be nearly as valuable. And a drug which promptly cured influenza would be equally or more valuable.

Another field in which cures may possibly be achieved at any time are for some of the most baffling chronic or relapsing maladies, such as rheumatoid arthritis and other rheumatic conditions, colitis, and multiple sclerosis. Total prevention would be best, but if we had remedies which permanently aborted these conditions as soon as they began, this would be almost as satisfactory. Immense research has already been devoted to them. And we have, regrettably, all too often been told that a 'breakthrough' has been achieved.

On the other hand, we can never expect to be able to cure the maladies due to degenerative arterial disease. The hope is that prevention will one day be achieved. We already have ways of ameliorating some kinds of arterial disease. Segments of obstructed leg arteries are replaced by lengths of vein, with marked improvement in the circulation to the leg. And segments of obstructed coronary arteries are similarly replaced, though with less convincing benefit. Further striking developments in this field are unlikely and I venture to prophesy that in future there will be a decline in the amount of coronary bypass surgery in the United States.

A huge proportion of the malaise of mankind is due to the disorders of the psyche. The prospects of spectacular advances in this field appear small. Much unhappiness is inextricably bound up with unsatisfactory relationships with other people, loneliness, monotonous work or no work at all, and dismal living conditions. Medicine can never put these matters right. Severe varieties of mental disorder, and schizophrenia in particular, are widely thought to be 'really' organic (see Chapter 2, p. 24), though I believe this view is false. We can already ameliorate to some extent the condition of schizophrenics by psychotropic drugs. It seems unlikely that there will be more than marginal improvement in the future. Analytical psychotherapy gives no proven benefit now; there is no reason to believe that it will ever give benefit in the future. The main hope for the improvement in the psychological state is from improvement in conditions of living and working.

PREVENTION

As everyone knows, many of the maladies of the affluent world are already 'preventible', but, with the possible exception of those related to tobacco, there is little prospect that they will in fact be prevented. The two groups of bodily maladies for which preventive measures are most eagerly desired are the cancers and the degenerative diseases.

To date the two means of preventing cancer have been the identification and subsequent removal of external factors and the excision of pre-cancerous lesions. Leaving aside carcinoma of the lung and other cancers related to tobacco, is there much hope that the other common cancers will be prevented by identifying external factors? A vast number of carcinogens, to which some people are exposed, have been identified and many workers in particular industries have died of various cancers in the past. Many of these dangerous carcinogens have already been removed. However, the great variation in the incidence of many cancers in different parts of the world (much of which cannot be explained on genetic grounds) suggests that there remain many more unidentified carcinogens. Doll concludes[2] (1977): 'it seems certain that environmental agents, of one sort or another, are responsible for the great majority of all cancers everywhere'.

Doll suggests that alcohol 'interacts with tobacco smoke and other agents to cause a variety of cancers of the upper respiratory and digestive tracts in a manner that is still not understood. It is also related ... to cancer of the liver ... and possibly to some cases of cancer of the pancreas and rectum ... it may account for some 5% of all fatal cancers in men'. Unfortunately, this incrimination of alcohol is unlikely to prevent much cancer, for obvious reasons.

There is suggestive evidence that some cancers may be related, not to the presence, but to the absence of certain factors. The lack of fibre in the diet of Western man may be associated with carcinoma of the lower bowel, as well as with diverticular disease and appendicitis. The mechanism of this association may be through the presence of anaerobic bacteroides. These are found especially in the alimentary tracts of those who eat low fibre, high meat and high fat diets. There are already good grounds for urging the public to eat more fibre and this is widely acceptable advice. The public are not so likely to follow advice to eat less meat and fat (though if these become increasingly expensive they may well do so).

There is as yet no clear proof that cancers in man are related to infections. But in view of the certain association between infections and some cancers in animals, it would be surprising if viruses never played any part in human cancer. Doll suggests that carcinomas of the nasopharynx and cervix uteri, Hodgkin's disease, childhood leukaemia and Burkitt's lymphoma may all be related to virus infections. The Epstein-Barr virus is probably the responsible organism in many cases. And carcinoma of the cervix uteri is commonly associated with infection by herpes virus, type II. The source of the infection is thought to be sexual promiscuity and the disease is rare in nuns. The hope here is that vaccines may be developed which prevent the viral infections, and in turn the malignant conditions.

Otherwise, we can reasonably hope that in future we will identify more and more carcinogens and other external factors. In principle the answer to the problem will then be simple, though in practice the public were only told 'the facts' they would cease from smoking. impossible. We should remember that when cigarette smoking was first shown to be so malign there were optimists who believed that if only the public were told 'the facts' they would cease from smoking.

The main example of the excision of pre-cancerous tissue in the hope of preventing cancer is carcinoma cervix uteri, though the evidence for the value of this procedure is conflicting (see Chapter 4, p. 62). There can also be no doubt that the removal of the colons of those affected by polyposis or by long-standing active ulcerative colitis is an effective means of preventing colonic carcinoma. But present medical knowledge indicates few if any other spheres where this kind of prevention is likely to be practicable.

An existing method by which cancer morbidity and mortality could be lessened is, it is widely thought, by discovering cancer 'early'. In fact, the value of this in practice appears small (see Chapter 4, p. 61). Neither is it likely that this method has much future potential.

DEGENERATIVE DISEASES

The biggest of all health problems in the affluent world is provided by the degenerative diseases. Arteriosclerosis is an essential feature of much of this disease; otherwise the condition which we would most of all like to prevent is non-arteriosclerotic senile dementia.

We can be confident that we shall never be able to prevent degerative processes; the most we can ever hope to do is to delay their onset or modify them. Moreover, genetic factors appear to play a large part here. In some families many members in turn develop senile dementia; in others the members retain their mental alertness until an advanced age. And the arteries of some very old people look like those of someone who is decades younger.

One can conceive that ultimately some kind of biochemical difference will be found between those who develop degenerative changes early and late. A way may then possibly be found of so changing the early subjects that they come to resemble the late ones.

The possibility that sometime we shall become able to live indefinitely in a state of hibernation, with all the bodily processes slowed down almost to zero, is often talked about. Thereby we would be able to obtain, if not immortality, a state not far removed from it. Anxious to know what the world will be like in 50 years time and how our grandchildren have developed and prospered, we would be able to go into hibernation and be re-activated 50 years later. But many people, myself included, believe that such a development would have the most unhappy consequences.

It is well to remember that degenerative processes can provide the best of all ways of dying. If someone has lived to an advanced age without mental deterioration and without serious bodily incapacity, what better end could be envisaged than to drop dead of a cardiac infarct, or to drop unconscious from a stroke and die within hours? Those fortunate to die in these ways are spared all the miseries of a long-term illness and their children are spared the horror of seeing a parent decline into an incontinent wreck. What worse disaster can there be than a massive but non-fatal stroke in a middle-aged person? He may live for years speechless, paralysed and incontinent, a burden to himself and everyone else.

What we would like to achieve is not, therefore, the prevention of degenerative processes, for that is impossible, but their postponement in those otherwise destined to develop them young and, in the case of strokes, the means of ensuring that all severe strokes are fatal. Unfortunately, we are never likely to achieve this second aim.

CONCLUSION

All the speculation about the future of medicine concerns technological discoveries - computers, more and more elaborate machines and more and more new drugs. But whatever the future holds, most of the time when people feel unwell and desire medical advice they are and probably always will be, affected by various minor physical ailments or by emotional problems or by both. And the most suitable person to deal with these patients will always be the General Practitioner who knows the patient and looks at him as a person against his background. Nothing can be more ludicrous than the idea that the doctor of first access will ever be replaced by some kind of computerized diagnostic machine which indicates that the patient should be referred to this or that specialist.

We should finally remember that people can and always will do far more for their own health than can the entire medical profession. When affected by most minor and some major ailments there is no point in seeing a doctor. We must hope that in future people will learn more about themselves and become better able to distinguish the occasions when they should and when they need not take medical advice.

SUMMARY

(1) In the affluent societies people have the power, by changing their habits, to improve greatly their state of health. Doctors have the power to reduce the cost of the curative services by a vast amount and simultaneously benefit patients. But the extrapolation of present trends suggests that many bad habits are still increasing and that doctors are increasingly wasteful. There seems little hope of a reversal in these trends in future.

(2) The degree of mechanization and computerization in medicine is bound to increase. But largely because single word or single phrase diagnoses are often absurd, the doctor will not be replaced by the machine. The best person to deal with most medical problems will always be the General Practitioner.

(3) Ever more sophisticated machines to take over the work of the bodily organs will be made. The amount of organ grafting will also increase, though it is doubtful whether the rejection problem will ever be solved.

(4) We shall probably never be able to cure most kinds of advanced disease. The most likely advances in curative medicine are in the treatment of viral illnesses and such baffling conditions as multiple sclerosis and rheumatoid arthritis. There is little prospect of improved treatment for psychological illness.

(5) The likeliest prospect of preventing cancer is by identifying and removing external factors. There is no prospect that most degenerative processes will be prevented, though they may be postponed.

(6) Whatever the future holds, the main reason for seeking medical advice will always be minor physical ailments or emotional problems. And people will always be able to do far more for their own health than the entire medical profession.

References

1. Seabord, G.T. (1968). *N. Y. State J. Med.*, **68,** 739
2. Doll, R. (1977). *J. R. Coll. Physicians,* **11,** 125

Index